W9-CEQ-500

ULTRALONGEVITY

ALSO BY MARK LIPONIS, MD

UltraPrevention (with Mark Hyman, MD)

ULTRA-
LONGEVITY

The **SEVEN-STEP PROGRAM** *for a*
YOUNGER, HEALTHIER YOU

MARK LIPONIS, MD

Little, Brown and Company

New York   Boston   London

For my parents, Charles and Bess Liponis, who taught
me the importance and value of love and family

Copyright © 2007 by Mark Liponis, MD

All rights reserved. Except as permitted under the U.S. Copyright Act of 1976, no part of this publication may be reproduced, distributed, or transmitted in any form or by any means, or stored in a database or retrieval system, without the prior written permission of the publisher.

Little, Brown and Company
Hachette Book Group USA
237 Park Avenue, New York, NY 10017
Visit our Web site at www.HachetteBookGroupUSA.com

First Edition: September 2007

This book is intended to supplement, not replace, the advice of a trained health professional. If you know or suspect that you have a health problem, you should consult a health professional. The author and publisher specifically disclaim any liability, loss, or risk, personal or otherwise, which is incurred as a consequence, directly or indirectly, of the use and application of any of the contents of this book.

Library of Congress Cataloging-in-Publication Data

Liponis, Mark.
    Ultralongevity : the seven-step program for a younger, healthier you / Mark Liponis. — 1st ed.
        p.   cm.
    Includes index.
    ISBN-13: 978-0-316-01728-2
    ISBN-10: 0-316-01728-0
    1. Longevity — Popular works.   2. Aging — Prevention — Popular works.
3. Nutrition — Popular works.   4. Self-Care, Health — Popular works.
I. Title.
    RA776.75.L564 2007
    613.2 — dc22   2007011225

10 9 8 7 6 5 4 3 2 1

Q-FF

Printed in the United States of America

CONTENTS

Introduction   3

The UltraLongevity Quiz: How Fast
   Are You Aging?   7

PART I   THE NEW SCIENCE OF THE
          IMMUNE SYSTEM

How the Immune System Works   23

The Players in the Immune System   33

How the Immune System Can Go Wrong   49

PART II   THE SEVEN-STEP ULTRALONGEVITY
          PROGRAM

Seven Steps to a Stronger Immune System   81

Step 1: Breathe   84

Step 2: Eat   99

Step 3: Sleep   124

Step 4: Dance   141

Step 5: Love   161

Step 6: Soothe   178

Step 7: Enhance   199

Contents

A Day in the Life of the
UltraLongevity Program   226

PART III   THE ULTRALONGEVITY EIGHT-DAY
MEAL PLAN

Eight Days to a Healthy Diet   233

Day 1   238

Day 2   245

Day 3   250

Day 4   255

Day 5   259

Day 6   264

Day 7   270

Day 8   276

Vegetarian Substitutions   281

Acknowledgments   287

Index   289

ULTRALONGEVITY

INTRODUCTION

THE LEGENDARY SPANISH explorer Juan Ponce de León supposedly spent the year 1513 searching for the Fountain of Youth. He wasn't the first person to look—stories of waters that restore youth to the aged have been popular throughout history. Such waters have been said to be located in Ethiopia, in distant Asia, in northern Europe, or many other places off the beaten path—for centuries people have explored, but without any luck.

After landing in the Americas, the Spanish began to hear tales from indigenous peoples about a fountain that could make adults young again. Excited at the prospect, they thought there was a strong chance these waters were located in what is now the state of Florida, or on the island of Bimini, just north of Cuba, which is where Ponce de León eventually sailed. He never did find the fountain there, but he did locate the Bahama Channel, the quickest route between Cuba and Europe. Ponce de León eventually was made a knight and later, governor of Florida. He died in 1521 at the relatively old age (for an explorer) of sixty-one.

His failure didn't stop countless other explorers, dreamers, alchemists, and adventurers from seeking a fountain of youth, whether in the form of water, a tonic, a pill, or anything else that would guarantee agelessness. No one, however, seemed to find it.

Then there's Laura, one of my patients. Over the last decade Laura has taken up, and mastered, both golf and tennis; whenever she comes to Canyon Ranch she manages to find a competitive game. She wasn't always so healthy, however. An asthmatic child, Laura visited the doctor frequently and was treated with shots of adrenaline numerous times even as a young adult. And in her early sixties she was diagnosed with breast cancer (she had a mastectomy).

But now Laura is in excellent health for someone her age, which is eighty-one (or twenty years older than Ponce de León was when he died). In fact, Laura is twenty years younger than her chronological age. Her heart purrs like a tuned engine. Tests of the elasticity of her arteries and heart rate variability are perfect. Her blood tests are all better than normal and into the optimal range.

Laura hasn't found the Fountain of Youth per se, but she is in on a secret that is helping her stay younger than everyone around her.

What is that secret? Laura has learned how to live in harmony with her immune system.

The theory guiding this new way of living stems from a growing body of research in a field that scientists and medical professionals are just beginning to understand: immunology, or the study of the immune system. What we are learning is that it isn't impossible—and, in fact, it might be quite probable—for humans to live to be well over one hundred years old.

Now, you might say that you don't *want* to live to one hundred. Who wants to spend years sitting in a wheelchair in the bleak hall of a cold, unpleasant nursing home? Meanwhile, your joints are arthritic, your bones brittle, your arteries clogged, your brain foggy, your lung capacity shrunk, and your muscle strength diminished. Your heart can't pump properly, you feel tired, and you're so constipated that having a good day means having a bowel movement.

Who wants to live to be one hundred if the above is an accurate description of aging?

But over the last few years medical science has learned that all the conditions just mentioned—all these terrible and painful signs of aging—are mainly caused by problems within the immune system.

In other words, the part of the body that was meant to defend us—the immune system—is actually turning on us, and causing us to age.

The fact that the immune system can turn dangerous has been known for some time. For a few decades now, medical science has understood that certain diseases, such as thyroid disease, multiple sclerosis, rheumatoid arthritis, ulcerative colitis, diabetes, and Crohn's disease, are diseases caused by the immune system, or what are known as autoimmune diseases.

These autoimmune diseases occur when the body is attacked by its own immune system. People who come down with autoimmune diseases tend to have highly overactive immune systems whose myriad weapons are attacking the body's own tissues instead of the various viruses and bacteria they are supposed to fight.

Scientists are beginning to understand that it is not just a few diseases that can be chalked up to this immune system hyperactivity. *It now appears that every disease of aging is associated with immune hyperactivity, and this hyperactivity is largely responsible for human aging itself.*

But just as we're realizing the nature of this medical issue, we are also starting to figure out ways to cope with it. This means that if you take the best possible care of your immune system and can prevent it from becoming overactive, you may well live to be more than one hundred years old—and be of healthy mind and body during every one of those years.

To put it another way, instead of feeling terrible in a nursing home, you can, like Laura, spend your life outdoors playing tennis, indoors learning new skills, or enjoying time with your loved ones—at any age.

If you can enhance your immune system, you won't live forever, but you may:

- Live more than a hundred years
- Be free from disease throughout your life
- Keep your brain sharp
- Be more physically fit
- Feel more energetic
- Be able to cope with stress
- Feel and stay younger than you ever imagined

Now, before you learn more about the immune system and its effects on your health, take the following test to see how much you already know.

THE ULTRALONGEVITY QUIZ: HOW FAST ARE YOU AGING?

EVER WONDER WHY people seem to age at different rates?

As you will soon learn, the speed of aging is determined by your immune system and, in fact, nearly all diseases are now thought to be caused by an immune system breakdown. Without a strong system, you will neither look healthy nor be healthy.

Following are twenty-one questions that touch on your lifestyle and your immune system. Answer them honestly, tally up your score, and discover how fast you are aging.

1. Do you need to lose ten pounds?
    a. Add 10 points if your weight is appropriate for your height.
    b. Add 5 points if you need to lose only ten pounds.
    c. Add no points if you need to lose more than ten pounds.

Carrying around extra weight is stressful—not just on your back and your joints, but on your immune system too. Besides causing you to be at higher risk for diseases such as diabetes, heart disease, and cancer, extra weight also can overstimulate your immune system.

One of the best ways to measure the extent of immune activation is the C-reactive protein (CRP) blood test—the higher your CRP levels, the more active your immune system is. A March 2006 article in the *Journal of the American Medical Association* (JAMA) showed that overweight women were eight to almost ten times more likely to have a hyperactive immune system—as demonstrated by higher levels of CRP than among women of healthy weight—even if they were physically active. Studies on men show similar results.

2. Do you smoke?
    a. Add 10 points if you rarely even smell smoke.
    b. Add 5 points if you're exposed to some secondhand smoke every day but you don't smoke.
    c. Add 2 points if you live with a smoker but don't smoke yourself.
    d. Add no points if you smoke.

Smoking is one guaranteed way to age your body faster. You know the effects—wrinkled skin, clogged arteries, emphysema, cancer, and impotence, to name just a few.

But the most important reason to stop smoking is that it over-stimulates the immune system, which in turn speeds up aging. A May 2005 study from the *American Heart Journal* revealed that smokers showed signs of high immune activation, including elevated CRP levels, as well as higher levels of macrophage-stimulating factors, which trigger our white blood cells to multiply, proliferate, and kill. (We'll talk more about that later.)

Even secondhand smoke causes immune activation. A February 2004 study in the *American Journal of Medicine* showed that people exposed to secondhand smoke at least three days a week had higher white blood counts, as well as higher CRP levels, than people not so exposed.

3. Do you live in one of the following metropolitan areas or cities: Birmingham (AL); Bakersfield, Fresno, Hanford-Corcoran, Los Angeles, Merced, Modesto, Sacramento, San

Diego, San Jose, Visalia (CA); Bridgeport (CT); Canton–Massillon, Cincinnati, Cleveland, Columbus, Steubenville–Weirton (OH–WV); Eugene–Springfield, Medford (OR); Harrisburg, Lancaster, Pittsburgh, Philadelphia (PA); Provo, Salt Lake City (UT); Seattle–Tacoma (WA); Charleston (WV); Huntington–Ashland (WV–KY–OH); Atlanta, Baltimore, Chicago, Detroit, Houston, Louisville, Knoxville, New York, Newark, St. Louis, or Washington, DC?

   a. Add 5 points if you live and work outside these areas.
   b. Add 2 points if you live in a rural or suburban area but often travel to the places listed frequently (i.e., weekly or more).
   c. Add no points if you live in one of these areas.

These are the forty most polluted metro areas or cities in the United States (not necessarily in order), measured by particulate air pollution and ozone. Breathing in polluted air activates your immune system into a constant defense mode that ages your body prematurely. A February 2006 study in the *American Journal of Respiratory and Critical Care Medicine* measured the day-to-day variations in CRP levels against the daily air pollution index. The study showed that CRP levels rose significantly approximately two days after subjects were exposed to particulate air pollution.

4. **Have you broken a sweat exercising in the past twenty-four hours?**
   a. Add 10 points if you break a sweat exercising at least four days a week.
   b. Add 5 points if you break a sweat at least twice a week.
   c. Add no points if you seldom exercise to a sweat.

Exercise helps deactivate the immune system in several ways. A report in the *American Journal of Cardiology* in January 2004 confirmed findings from research in 2002, published in *Circulation* and in *Epidemiology*, which showed an inverse relationship between exercise and CRP: exercise lowers CRP levels. It's no surprise that exercise has been proven to prevent just about every disease and reduce the effects of aging.

5. What was your birth weight?
   a. Add 4 points if you weighed more than 8½ pounds but less than 10 pounds at birth.
   b. Add 2 points if you weighed between 7 and 8½ pounds.
   c. Add no points if you weighed less than 7 pounds or more than 10 pounds at birth.

Research shows that smaller babies (5½ to 6 pounds) have prematurely aged immune systems, while larger babies (up to 9½ pounds) lead longer lives with less disease. Lower birth weight has been linked to higher levels of CRP and immune activation in adult life. In the recent MIDSPAN Family Study, a large-scale, long-term survey conducted in Scotland, researchers found that in the range between 5½ and 9½ pounds, CRP levels in adults were inversely proportional to their birth weight, and that within that range every kilogram (2.2 pounds) at birth meant 11 percent lower CRP levels in adulthood.

6. Have you taken an antibiotic medication in the past year?
   a. Add 4 points if you can't remember the last time you took an antibiotic.
   b. Add 2 points if you've taken a course of antibiotics no more than ten times in your life.
   c. Add no points if you generally take a course of antibiotics every year or more often.

Antibiotic use prematurely ages the immune system and is linked to a number of health effects, including heart disease, allergies, asthma, and even breast cancer. Frequent antibiotic use is a sign of someone whose immune system is often in battle mode, fighting an infection but also wreaking havoc on his or her health in the process.

A study published in *Chest* in March 2006 demonstrated that babies exposed to even one course of antibiotics in the first year of life faced twice as much risk of developing asthma as non-exposed babies, and that risk increased with each successive course of antibiotics.

7. Do you have older siblings?
    a. Add 4 points if you have older brothers or sisters.
    b. Add no points if you're an only or oldest child.

Research suggests that only children or oldest siblings are often more prone to allergies, eczema, asthma, and other allergic disorders, which are indicative of an overactive immune system.

A review of fifty-three existing studies, published in the *Journal of Epidemiology and Community Health* in 2002, showed a strong and consistent relationship between the number of siblings and allergies, asthma, wheezing, and hay fever, with the risk increasing with fewer siblings.

8. Is your belly bigger than your hips?
    a. Add 10 points if your hips are bigger (yeah!).
    b. Add 2 points if your belly and hip measurements are the same.
    c. Add no points if your belly is bigger than your hips.

Your hip measurement should be more than your waist measurement, at least 10 percent more for men and 20 percent more for women. Carrying extra inches around the middle of your body is an immune system disorder and is linked with premature aging. This rule holds true even for people who are not overweight. A study from Brigham and Women's Hospital in Boston, published in *Epidemiology* in November 2003, showed that even when weight was normal, having a waist measurement as large as one's hip measurement was linked with higher levels of immune hyperactivity.

9. Did you floss your teeth today?
   a. Add 2 points if you flossed today.
   b. Add 1 point if you did not but often do.
   c. Add no points if you seldom or never floss.

Yes, floss. Flossing helps reduce plaque buildup in the teeth and gums. This plaque is a thick coating of nasty bacteria that creates a constant struggle with your immune system. High levels of plaque are linked with an overactive immune system and a doubled risk of cardiovascular disease. Research from the *Archives of Internal Medicine* (October 2000) found that periodontal disease doubled the risk of stroke in adults over twenty-five. Also, according to a study from the Harvard Dental School and Brigham and Women's Hospital (published in the February 2001 *Journal of the American College of Cardiology*), higher rates of heart attacks, death from cardiovascular causes, and stroke were found in people with periodontal disease.

10. Have you made love in the past week?
   a. Add 5 points if you have a good love life.
   b. Add 3 points if you have a fair love life.
   c. Add 1 point if you're frustrated with your love life
      (at least you know what a love life is!).

Just what you were waiting for: sex is good for you. Well, actually it's not just sex; it's loving and feeling loved. Little quiets down a revved-up immune system better than knowing someone else loves you, and vice versa. When you love and feel loved, not only does everything seem better in the world, it is better in your body too.

11. Did you tell a funny joke to your friends today that made them laugh?
  a. Add 2 points if you made someone laugh.
  b. Add 1 point if someone made you laugh.
  c. Add no points if you can't remember laughing today.

Okay, this is a bit of a trick question. If you answered yes, we know two things: you have friends, and you have a sense of humor (plus good delivery). What's important here is camaraderie and laughter. Both are rejuvenating to the immune system. "Laughter is the best medicine" is not just an old chestnut. Laughter sends a signal to the immune system to chill out.

12. Did you grow up with a dog?
  a. Add 2 points if you grew up with a dog.
  b. Add 1 point if you grew up with any pet.
  c. Add no points if you never had animals.

Besides being a best friend, a pet plays an important role in supporting your immune system. Dogs and cats (and some other pets) create contact with most of the harmless germs our immune system needs to get to know as it develops in our childhood (however, people should be a little more careful with cats, as cats tend to cause more allergies than dogs). Without exposure to the right germs, your immune system runs amok and starts reacting to all kinds of things it shouldn't, such as pollen, grass, hay, dander, and/or mold, leading to allergies, asthma, and skin rashes.

13. Have you had a massage in the last month?
    a. Add 2 points if you were massaged.
    b. Add 1 point if you massaged someone else.
    c. Add no points if you haven't done either.

Talk about being relaxed. Having every tired muscle rubbed for an hour while your brain takes a holiday is good medicine. Relaxing touch combined with a release of muscle pain goes a long way toward reducing tension in your immune system too. Massage has been shown to reduce activation of the immune system, and it feels good besides.

14. Do you eat more than three times a day? (If more than one answer applies, pick the one that applies best.)
    a. Add 5 points if you're a grazer and almost never overeat.
    b. Add 3 points if you skip a meal now and then but usually eat three meals a day and don't often overeat.
    c. Add 0 points if you eat large meals and usually feel stuffed afterward.

Eating three meals a day is no longer considered the healthiest meal pattern. Meals are one of the biggest stresses on your immune system. Worse, pooling all of your day's calories into just one or two large meals is excessively stressful on your immune system. The bigger the meal, the higher the levels of CRP and interleukin-6 and the more activated your immune system—especially after a fatty meal. Grazing, or eating several smaller meals, is a better strategy than eating just two or three larger meals a day.

15. Do you take vitamins?
    a. Add 4 points if you take a multivitamin an hour before your biggest meal of the day.

  b. Add 2 points if you take a multivitamin every day, but
     not before your biggest meal.
  c. Add no points if you don't take a multivitamin.

Taking a multivitamin daily reduces stress on the immune system and slows aging. In fact, it has been shown to reduce CRP
levels significantly, according to a study in the *American Journal of
Medicine* in December 2003.

However, if you're like most people, you probably take your
multivitamin first thing in the morning. Your multivitamin is actually best taken about an hour before your biggest meal of the day,
when it acts to help reduce the immune activation that occurs after
a meal. Research reported in *Circulation* in July 2003 showed that
taking antioxidant vitamins A, C, E, and beta carotene before dinner prevented the rise in CRP observed after a meal.

16. **Have you raised your voice in anger over the past twenty-
    four hours?**
    a. Add 5 points if you can honestly say that you rarely get
       angry at anything.
    b. Add 1 point if you felt angry but didn't yell.
    c. Add no points if you've raised your voice today.

Be honest. Yelled at your kids? Your spouse? At the office?
At the store? At anyone? How about your dog? Even when your
voice gets a little edgy, it's a sign of inner hostility. Hostility and
anger are powerful emotions that tell your immune system you're
geared up for a fight. Translation: Get ready to be hurt by an overactive immune system. In a study from Duke University's Behavioral Sciences Department published in *Psychosomatic Medicine* in
September 2004, a higher degree of anger and hostility was found
to predict higher CRP levels.

17. Do you feel anxious during the day?

   a. Add 2 points if you're just occasionally anxious.
   b. Add no points if you're anxious nearly all the time.
   c. If you're never anxious, add no points, because lying isn't good for your immune system either.

Nervous? Sweaty palms? Outright scared? Or even just kind of flustered? Your immune system isn't happy when you get nervous. Anxiety sends a loud and clear message—you feel threatened. That's exactly when your defense system kicks in. Frequent anxiety ages you prematurely.

In the wake of 9/11, Israeli researchers assessed the effect of chronic anxiety on health and immune function by studying CRP levels in 721 men and 431 women. Especially in women, fear of terrorism was associated with elevated CRP, indicating activation of the immune system.

18. Ever feel down in the dumps? Blue? Sad? Outright despairing?

   a. Add 5 points if you're generally positive and optimistic.
   b. Add 2 points if you've felt depressed more than once in the past month.
   c. Add no points if you often feel depressed.

Of the three most dangerous emotions (hostility, anxiety, and despair), despair is probably the worst; it tells your immune system that you are not just anxious, but that you've also given up. Despair and depression have been linked with all sorts of conditions, from heart disease to brain decline to osteoporosis. If it's a frequent condition, depression clearly needs treatment. Many studies have now shown this, including a hallmark one reported in the October 1996 New England Journal of Medicine that linked depression with osteoporosis. Since then, research has also coupled depression with increased incidence of diabetes, heart disease, stroke, and cancer.

19. Did you sleep well last night?
   a. Add 5 points if you almost always sleep like a baby.
   b. Add 3 points if you usually sleep like a baby.
   c. Add 1 point if you often don't get enough sleep.
   d. Add no points if you're always tired and you still don't seem to get enough sleep.

When you sleep, your immune system can finally relax, recharge, and repair. It can't do this during the day—it's too busy defending you. This is why it's difficult to sleep when you're sick, because your immune system is so busy. All kinds of repair processes occur during sleep, while sleep deprivation is an important cause of immune hyperactivity as proven by many studies, including one reported in the February 2004 *Journal of the American College of Cardiology* showing that both short-term and chronic sleep deprivation led to elevated CRP levels.

20. Do you sing? Hum? Often have a song running through your head?
   a. Add 2 points if you play an instrument or sing every day.
   b. Add 1 point if you often listen to your home music system or portable music player.
   c. Add no points if you couldn't care less about music. It won't help you, but it probably won't age you either.

Music soothes more than the savage beast—it soothes your immune system. Bach, Beethoven, Earl Scruggs, or Eminem will do. Research on babies in a neonatal intensive care unit showed that when recorded lullabies were played, babies had better oxygen levels, fewer infections, and shorter hospital stays (*Pediatric Nursing*, 1998).

21. What time of the year were you born?
    a. Add 2 points if you were born in the spring.
    b. Add 1 point if you were born in the winter or summer.
    c. Add no points if you were born in the fall.

No, this is not about astrology. Research by Caleb Finch and Eileen Crimmins, as reported in the September 17, 2004, issue of *Science,* showed that, on average, people born in the spring seem to age a bit more slowly and tend to live three to six months longer than people born in the fall.

The explanation may lie in the seasonal variation in birth weight and its impact on our immune system (the opposite pattern is seen in people born in the southern hemisphere).

KEY

If your score is:

80–100: You are aging like a redwood tree, living in harmony with your calm and secure immune system. There's no need for it to be overactive, and peace reigns in your bloodstream. But there's always room for improvement. Read on and learn how to slow the aging process even further.

60–79: You are aging like a giant tortoise. Your immune system is your friend and has little interest in attacking you—at the moment. It's possible to improve upon your success and make your immune system work even better. There are several steps you can take to slow down the aging process and live a longer, healthier life. Learn on!

40–59: You are aging like the average human, which isn't bad, but you could be aging much more slowly while at the same time reducing your risk of getting sick. Knowledge is power, so here's your chance to learn how to slow the aging process and prevent disease. There are many things you can do right now to improve your immune function, starting with the right mind-set: believe that you have the power to change your health and your aging speed.

20–39: You are aging like a speeding bullet, heading for a dreaded disease—if you don't already have one. This score calls for immediate action to stop this process. You probably should skip ahead to the UltraLongevity program in Part II; you can always come back and read Part I once you've taken the first steps to gain control of your immune system.

1–19: You are aging like a dinosaur (nearly extinct already). To score this low, you must be trying to hasten your own demise. But the mere fact that you're reading this book means there's still hope. Pause. Take a breath. Affirm to yourself that you are worth taking care of. And read on. This is the start of a whole new you, and you are in the driver's seat. Even people who score this low can, and have, changed their lives for the better!

PART I

THE NEW SCIENCE OF THE IMMUNE SYSTEM

HOW THE IMMUNE
SYSTEM WORKS

AGING IS AN autoimmune disease. It is caused by your own immune system attacking you.

Yes, that's correct. Aging is not a natural result of living too many years. There are many examples in nature of organisms that can live indefinitely without displaying any signs of aging whatsoever. But as you will learn, unlike humans, these organisms lack a complex immune system.

According to the latest findings in medical science, all of the conditions that we consider part of aging—including arthritis, osteoporosis, Alzheimer's disease, cancer, stroke, heart disease, poor brain functioning, weak lungs, and diabetes—are not simply the result of getting older, but are conditions caused by an overactive immune system.

What this means is that, for the first time in history, medicine now has a plausible and coherent theory of aging that is fully supported by medical research.

IT ISN'T JUST ABOUT COUNTING BIRTHDAYS

If you took the aging quiz, you've already learned that aging isn't simply about being thirty, or forty-five, or sixty. These are just numbers indicative of years that have passed. We are all going to get older, in terms of moments spent on earth. Clocks keep ticking. Time passes. That doesn't necessarily mean we are all aging at the same rate. Year by year, some of us are aging much more slowly than others.

So if aging isn't the number of years you've lived, what is it? *Aging represents the cumulative changes in an organism, organ, tissue, or cell that eventually lead to a decrease in function and ultimately death. Furthermore, this decrease in function is primarily brought on by an immune system that is highly overactive.*

This means that decreased function of the skin, bones, heart, nerves, lungs, kidneys, and all of the other organs throughout your body is caused by an immune system that is far more active than it should be.

Think about it. Function is more important than chronological age. We don't really care about the actual age of the heart, for instance, as long as it is functioning well. Similarly, we wouldn't care if we were 150 years old if all of our organs were operating at peak performance.

And what causes this loss of function that leads to aging? The immune system.

Now, how could that be? We think of our immune system as our friend. Shouldn't it be helping us? And how could our immune system cause us to age?

To understand this paradox, you need to understand two things: the function of our immune system, and how we age.

As mentioned, aging is synonymous with deteriorating organs and organ function. Our brains lose neurons and brainpower, our heartbeat weakens, our lung capacity drops, our joints get stiff, and our bones get thinner. You know, or can guess, the rest: bladder shrinking, muscles fading, eyes dimming, skin thinning, general overall decline, and eventually, disease leading to death.

Despite what you've often heard, people don't actually die of old age. They die of heart failure, or lung failure, or kidney failure, or liver failure, or brain failure, or sometimes all of the above. So aging is really a progressive decline in the function of our organs until they lose so much function disease arises.

But disease is not necessarily a feature of getting older. It's not uncommon for people to be quite old without any sign of disease or diminished organ function.

Disease is not programmed into our genes. Actually, disease and aging itself—the decrease in organ function—both result from a hyperactive immune system.

Our immune system is a complex and highly evolved system with a single goal: defense. It evolved in a dangerous world filled with threats from innumerable attackers and today is truly miraculous in its capabilities and complexity. It's amazing to think how powerful and diverse a system it is, able to protect us from a bewildering number of possible dangers.

But as humans continue to evolve and adapt to a changing environment, the trade-off between protection and an overactive immune system is increasingly important.

Today we have vaccines, antibiotics, better hygiene, and early detection and preventive measures that reduce the likelihood of the serious infections that our immune system has evolved to handle. As a result, people in the developed world are no longer dying as often from these infections as they are from conditions such as heart disease, diabetes, or Alzheimer's.

We are entering a time in human evolution when our immune systems are becoming too powerful to allow us to reach our full potential life span. Thankfully, humans are adaptable, resourceful, and intelligent. We are learning how to gain control over our immune system—by applying what we've learned through scientific research, we will be able to extend our longevity so we can live to what is now considered extreme old age, without disease or decrepitude.

Now, I don't mean that humans will ever change the fact that we grow chronologically older every year. We are not talking about immortality. But we are learning how to change the *nature* of how we grow older, because we are learning how to maintain the level of our organ function.

The fact is that not *all* aging is caused by the immune system alone. Factors such as gravity and exposure to atmospheric radiation have a deleterious effect, causing injuries to our bodies that we don't yet have protection against. Perhaps someday we will wear antigravity suits and live in sanitized cities surrounded by bubbles. Until then, we will not be able to combat all of the external causes of aging.

It also seems likely that to some degree, aging may be genetically preprogrammed into humans. In other words, we might well be predetermined to grow old. However, just as we now know little about this, it's also possible that as we learn more, we may be able to combat even our own genes.

But even with the effects of gravity and radiation, and the genetically preprogrammed effects that create senescence, medical science now believes that humans should be able to live to 150 years old.

You might not think you want to live that long, because you imagine that life after 80 is terrible. Yet we've learned that people who have excellent immune systems and live long lives flourish long after the age of 80. The oldest human on record was Frenchwoman Jeanne Calment, who lived to 122 years old. Calment learned how to fence at 85, rode a bike at 100, and released a rap CD at 121.

Bear in mind that for decades, science has been extending the maximum life span. Like a bullish stock market, the numbers keep rising. Once it was 90, then 100, then 110, then 120; today we're past that. It's not clear how far we can go because we don't have proof. But we do know it is surely longer than 122 years, and we expect many people who are alive today to surpass that number.

When asked how they live so long, many of the record-breaking respondents credit oddities such as a daily glass of whiskey, a taste for chocolate, or a sexual appetite. Whether or not there's any legitimacy to these claims, something else is actually at work, and that's the immune system. What's now clear is that people who live to be over 100 years old have immune systems that are able to resist overstimulation and hyperactivity.

I fully believe that the latest scientific research shows that the effects of aging are mediated through the immune system, and that the best way to live a long and healthy life is to get your immune system functioning at its peak.

WHAT IS THE IMMUNE SYSTEM?

The immune system is one of the most complicated systems science has ever encountered. This section of the book provides a brief explanation of how it works, and what happens when it isn't working well. You don't need to know all of this in order to follow the seven simple steps presented in Part II, but I've always felt that a dose of knowledge is a good thing: you'll understand more about the UltraLongevity recommendations, and you'll know more about why they were made.

The immune system is a collection of cells and organs in your body that defend you against the world. In other words, your immune system protects you from the constant invaders and trespassers your body encounters every day, whether these are dangerous viruses, lethal bacteria, toxic parasites, or less harmful particles that enter the body.

It is a remarkably complex system, more so than any other in the human body, including the brain, yet it is not well understood. One of the problems in grasping its entirety is that the immune system is not made up of one single organ. Unlike the brain, the heart, or any other organ upon which you can (literally) put your finger, the immune system isn't localized. It doesn't exist in one place. It comprises both organs and cells, and it exists nearly everywhere in your body.

HOW DID THE IMMUNE SYSTEM DEVELOP?

The immune system does not exist in all animals—lower organisms, for example, don't possess one, and yet many of these creatures seem capable of living indefinitely, without showing signs of aging. The simplest of these beings, viruses, are ostensibly immortal; recently, bacteria trapped inside prehistoric amber were found to be alive and estimated at approximately 250 million years old.

Numerous plants seem to live forever also—science has found eighty-thousand-year-old quaking aspens and forty-three-thousand-year-old King's Holly. And recent discoveries of massive underground fungi show these organisms to be at least two thousand years old—with no signs of aging whatsoever.

Many simple sea creatures such as sea urchins and snails also display no hints of aging; older specimens don't die any faster than younger ones.

The immune system doesn't appear in the evolutionary ladder until organisms become more complicated. We don't know why it developed, but although this may sound strange, it's plausible that at some point in the very distant past, two wholly different kinds of creatures united to form a single, more adaptable and powerful new being. Maybe it was some slime mold that absorbed a paramecium, or a jellyfish that engulfed a prehistoric amoeba, but it's possible that this union produced an advantageous combination.

In fact, the jellyfish seems to be the first creature on the evolutionary ladder to possess a rudimentary immune system. Perhaps eons ago a jellyfish absorbed a certain kind of amoeba that then acted symbiotically as a defense system for its host, attacking and gobbling up any would-be invaders such as bacteria, molds, or viruses.

In the meantime, the jellyfish provided a safe environment in which the amoeba could flourish, giving it an ample supply of food and nutrients. Plus, there was no real chance of rejection, since jellyfish, lacking an immune system, did not have an internal structure that could toss the amoeba out. Hence a partnership may have been born.

From then on, subsequent reproduction would have duplicated both organisms' DNA, and a brand-new being would have been created, now with its own fledgling immune system. Over the next many, many millions of years, evolution could then have refined and developed the system into a more complex, efficient, and robust one.

Of course this is speculation, but it's not out of the realm of possibility. And if you were actually able to see how the cells of our immune system act and react, seemingly of their own volition, the theory becomes very believable.

THE IMMUNE SYSTEM'S JOB

The immune system has two important tasks.

The first is defensive. As mentioned, the immune system must protect you every moment of the day and night, going into battle against all of the potentially harmful intruders constantly attacking you.

The second task is more surprising. The immune system must store memories—and not just a few. It must place in its memory bank every battle it has ever fought, as well as every intruder it has ever met. Otherwise, your immune system would eventually fail to protect you.

After all, if it never learned anything from its previous battles, it would be fighting the same wars over and over, fruitlessly taking on intruders that turn out to be harmless, or not remembering which weapons to use to handle which serious invaders.

GROG

To help us understand the immune system's place in history, let's pretend we're in the Pleistocene era, where one of my patients is Grog, a Cro-Magnon man.

Grog is having a tough day. In fact, he's having a tough life. The Cro-Magnons lived between forty thousand and ten thousand years ago, and they all had a difficult time—it wasn't easy being prehistoric. Cro-Magnons' remains are remarkable for their enormous number of broken bones and infections.

Grog, like most of his tribe, spends his day hunting, which means running on the ground with bare feet, and he is constantly coming down with injuries. Today he has a terrible infection, which is why he's seeing me.

In taking his family history, I learn there's not much good news. Grog's mother died giving birth to Grog's brother when she was eighteen. Grog's father fell into a canyon and broke his back; because no one in the tribe could save him, he was left to die.

Grog's tribe is vaguely aware of the concept of infections because they're so frequent. But they don't have any idea where they come from, what they are, or how to cope with them. However, the tribe buries its dead, and it seems as though they do this in part

Humans exist in an eat-or-be-eaten world. Everything that lives is predator or prey. This process occurs on many levels, both outside and inside our bodies.

We humans think of ourselves as predators, but we are also prey, under the persistent threat of billions of invisible microbes whose primary intent is attacking, and potentially killing, us. To fight them off, we have developed a highly evolved and complex system of defense.

To understand this fully, consider a relevant topic from today's headlines: homeland security.

because they realize that leaving bodies around to rot will spread disease.

Grog himself is a veritable walking infection—he has boils on his skin, an abscess on his jaw, bad teeth, and terrible breath. His white blood count is very high because his body is always fighting off infections; he also has a high C-reactive protein (CRP) level, indicating a high level of immune system activity.

One thing Grog doesn't have: allergies. Dirt is ground into every pore of his body, but because of this, his immune system has never had time to develop allergies. Dirt can be good—it gives our immune system something to do, relieving the boredom of the job.

What Grog does have right now is an overwhelming infection. While he was running in the woods after a deer, he stepped on a sharp rock, cut his sole, walked through the mud, and now has germs in his foot. The infection is crawling up his leg into his lymph nodes and into his groin. Now he can't fend for himself.

There's nothing I or any other doctor can do for him, because in Grog's time the only possible remedy is to try to drain the infection. For Grog, it's far too little too late, and like most Cro-Magnons in his situation, Grog will soon die from an overwhelming infection that has gone systemic.

Our country is susceptible to all manner of attacks from terrorists: from the air and the sea, from chemical and nuclear weapons, from contaminated water supplies and poisonous gases. To protect ourselves, we've created a very complex defense system for homeland security. We have a huge border that we patrol regularly. We have information agencies that constantly gather intelligence. We have weapons ready at all times to thwart invaders.

There is no single line of defense. Instead, we try to protect our country from all means of attack.

The same is true inside our bodies. We must protect our body, which is, in effect, our homeland. To do this, our immune system has a complex set of duties similar to those of the U.S. Department of Homeland Security. It has a huge exterior border to patrol, as well as a large interior space to protect. Threats to our bodies include attacks from outside and within, from the air we breathe, the food we eat, the water we drink, and contact with other people. We are subject to chemical exposures and radiation. Our immune system must protect us from every line of attack.

Outside invaders can assault us not only through the most obvious frontier, the skin, but by crossing other borders, including internal organs such as the lungs, gut, digestive tract, nose, throat, and so on.

These borders are subject to attack from any number of different threats, including bacteria or viruses, allergens, parasites, yeasts, molds, toxic chemicals, noxious fumes, and even dangerous proteins such as prions.

To win the battles against these terrorists, our immune system is armed with dozens of specialized weapons wielded by various combatants. Scientists have already identified at least twenty different types of immune cells, and new ones are still being discovered. Despite the numbers and types of different cells and their complexity, there are only a few you need to know about in order to understand the most important ways in which your immune system works to protect you.

THE PLAYERS IN THE IMMUNE SYSTEM

INSIDE YOU ARE more than thirty different organs, which include more than two hundred different cell types and about 100 trillion cells. Each organ is patrolled by your immune system, which is constantly performing surveillance for possible threats. Following are some of the major players.

BONE MARROW

Bone marrow, the reddish-looking material inside nearly every bone in the human body, is where all of the blood cells are produced.

Inside the marrow, on an inner framework, lie the bone marrow stem cells. These cells are constantly dividing, producing huge numbers of cells that turn into red and white blood cells.

The bone marrow stem cells continue to divide, even as they keep making red and white blood cells. And just as a couple of million are being produced every second, the same number are being gobbled up and destroyed in the spleen, which is, in effect, the cells' decommissioning center. The spleen is where blood cells are taken out of circulation once they've completed their useful life cycle (see below).

This process—birth in the bone marrow, death in the spleen—should be evenly balanced. If it isn't, you will be prone to a blood disorder. For example, if your system is destroying more red blood cells than it's making, you'll become anemic, which will make you feel tired and appear pale. If you're making more than you are destroying, you'll become polycythemic, or suffer from blood that is overcrowded with red blood cells.

Once the cells form in the bone marrow, they remain there and mature, at which time they exit and enter the bloodstream. There they circulate, the red cells carrying oxygen and carbon dioxide, and the white cells patrolling for invaders.

THE THYMUS

The thymus, located in front of your windpipe in the upper chest region, is the most mysterious organ in your homeland.

In infants, the thymus is, relatively speaking, huge. It grows until about puberty and then starts to shrink. By old age, the thymus has almost completely disappeared.

The thymus serves the role of a kind of boot camp for the white blood cells called T cells—it's where these cells go to mature. The thymus is especially active early in life because, during youth, T cells are constantly being exposed to new things, from new proteins in your diet to new germs. These T cells need to have a place to congregate, share information, and learn about threats and attacks.

For example, let's say one of the cells in your immune system comes in contact with a foreign invader. It now has to communicate that information to other cells so they can become aware of the invader too. The thymus is where this information is shared and training occurs.

Why does the thymus later atrophy? Science doesn't know for certain, but as you grow older, your immune system has less to learn. So the current thinking is that there may be less need for a large thymus as we age. But although the thymus is not as big or as active as it was when we were young, the smaller thymus is still able to help train T cells well into our eighties, nineties, and beyond.

THE SPLEEN

Another important training center and meeting ground for the immune system is the spleen. This large organ, about the size of your fist, is located on the left side of your belly, tucked under your ribs.

The spleen is a common meeting place for all the immune system's cells. Blood routes to the spleen, where the cells circulate and mingle, allowing them to tell each other what they've learned, what they've seen, what they've killed, and what antibodies they've made.

The heart pumps the blood around the body about once every minute, which means each blood cell might find itself in the spleen about 1,400 times a day. That's a great many trips.

The spleen is also important because it's where the body decides if a red or a white blood cell has gotten too old. Once the decision is made, the cell is decommissioned and disassembled and its building blocks are recycled.

You can live without a spleen; if it ruptures, the liver can take over its functions. Still, if your spleen is removed or no longer works, your immunity becomes impaired; people without a spleen are more susceptible to infections.

LYMPHATIC SYSTEM

Nearly everyone knows about the bloodstream: it's a road map of blood vessels that allow our blood to circulate through our body. But few people realize that another important, and completely different, circulatory system exists in the body—the lymphatic system, which circulates our lymph.

Lymph is a clear fluid that travels through your body, cleaning your tissues and keeping them nourished. Just as blood circulates back to the heart through our veins, lymph must also be recycled and return to the heart, which it does through the lymphatic system.

The lymphatic system is something of a secondary transportation system for your homeland troops. Like the circulatory system, it is composed of a series of vessels and tubes. The major difference between the circulatory and the lymphatic systems is that the latter lacks a pump to move the fluid it carries. For the blood, that pump is the heart. For lymph, the flow back to the heart is achieved through a more passive process involving muscle contractions and gravity.

You may have noticed that your feet swell during a long journey on an airplane or in a car. This is due to lack of movement; your muscles haven't been able to circulate lymph, so because of gravity, it collects at the lowest part of your body—your feet.

You also may be aware of a condition known as edema, which is swelling that results from a collection of lymph. Edema occurs when excess lymph fluid cannot be returned back into circulation.

The bloodstream is extensive, branching out from its main trunk, the aorta, as well as smaller arteries, arterioles, capillaries, veins, and venules, but there is still a large portion of our tissues the capillaries can't reach.

Here is where the lymph comes into play. Nutrients such as glucose (blood sugar) must be helped so they can reach and nourish each and every cell, including those the bloodstream can't reach. That happens via the lymph fluid, which bathes and nourishes all of the body's tissues. And once those nutrients have been used, the fluid must be recycled or your body would swell up like the Michelin tire man.

Along the course of the lymphatic system are way stations known as lymph nodes. These are outposts whose sentries make sure nothing passes through the lymphatic channels that shouldn't. The lymphatic system could provide easy and direct access for a germ or microbe to our heart and bloodstream, so to prevent that from happening, lymphocytes (T cells and B cells) aggregate in lymph nodes, waiting for something bad to pass by. When they spot that something, the node cells attack before it can venture into the heart and bloodstream.

When a problem is stirring in your body, the lymph nodes become enlarged. For example, if you have swollen glands in the neck, your nodes may have found some virus that landed in the back of the throat and is trying to gain access to the lungs or bloodstream. Lymph nodes responding to some infection can become swollen almost anywhere: in the groin, neck, chest, abdomen, and so on.

WHITE BLOOD CELLS

Probably the most important cells of our immune system, as well as the best-known and the most numerous, are the white blood cells. This term distinguishes them from the red blood cells, the disklike cells responsible for carrying oxygen and carbon dioxide from our lungs throughout the rest of the body.

Most people probably think of white blood cells simply as formless globules floating through our bloodstream, randomly patrolling for microbes. But our white blood cells are very purposeful and deliberate in their surveillance, and there are actually many different types of white blood cells, each with specialized functions. And these white blood cells are found not just in the blood, but throughout our bodies—in each of our organs, from the brain to the liver to the lungs, as well as throughout the lymphatic system.

The first line of immune cells are the lymphocytes. *Cyte* means "cell," so lymphocytes are the lymph or lymphatic cells. The ones you most need to know about are the B lymphocytes (better known as B cells) and the T lymphocytes (better known as *T cells*).

B CELLS

B cells were so named because they were first studied in the bursa of Fabricius, an organ unique to birds. In humans, B cells actually originate in the bone marrow.

The B cells have two major jobs: they maintain a memory database, and they create complex protein structures that are used as weapons against threats and invaders. These complex structures are called antibodies, about which more is coming.

B cells keep a record of every single interaction your immune system has ever had. This means that within your body, a record of every germ and virus you've ever encountered, every protein you've ever eaten, every piece of pollen you've ever inhaled, has been stored in a memory bank—not in your brain, but in your immune system. Think about it: for each of these interactions, there is a B cell floating around inside your body that has retained a memory of the encounter.

Your immune system's memory is, in some ways, more impressive than your brain's. Most of us can only evoke faint memories from early childhood. Your immune system, however, remembers your first vaccination, which probably occurred in the earliest days of your life. Research now suggests that your immune system even stores memories from when you were still developing in your mother's womb.

Shortly after birth, you were probably immunized with vaccines for diphtheria, tetanus, and pertussis (whooping cough). Although the memory of that immunization may fade somewhat, and a booster may be needed to remind your immune system, some remnant of that memory lasts a lifetime.

These stored memories are critically important for your survival; they are what make you immune to becoming sick more than once from certain illnesses.

For example, after a bout of chicken pox in childhood, you

become immune—you usually can't catch chicken pox again as an adult. Likewise, after being immunized with a shot for tetanus, you won't succumb to the bacterial infection that causes tetanus. Your B cells now have the memory stored away and prevent you from coming down with the disease.

A memory of exposure to prior threats is crucial because it allows your immune system to respond more quickly and effectively to serious threats if you are reexposed. Without such a memory, and a rapid response, exposure to ailments such as tetanus or diphtheria could be fatal.

It's also important for your immune system to remember prior contacts and exposures even if they're not potentially lethal, as it makes your immune system less likely to cause an overwhelming reaction when encountering nonlethal microbes. If, for example, your immune system overreacted every time you ate a particular food, or breathed in a particular pollen, you would forever exist in a state of immune hyperactivity and unnecessary battle.

One example of an overreaction by our immune system is an allergy, which can trigger serious problems like asthma or even anaphylaxis, which can be lethal. We'll talk more about this later.

B cells possess another important function. They make antibodies, whose role in your internal homeland security is similar to that of the U.S. Army Corps of Engineers. Here B cells work closely with T cells to build complex mechanical and chemical structures that act as deadly weapons to neutralize invaders.

Antibodies are complex proteins manufactured to exact specifications. Each antibody is built by the B cells to neutralize one specific invader. Medical science does not yet fully understand the way in which these antibodies are made. What is known is that B cells team up with macrophages in order to create them.

First, what is a macrophage? *Phage* comes from the Greek *phagon*, meaning "to eat." *Macro*, from the Greek *macron*, means "big." Thus a macrophage is a "big eater."

Macrophages constantly patrol the body, which means they can be considered your body's military police, or MPs. The MPs are constantly on the lookout, in every organ in your body. Always moving, they crawl between the trillions of cells in all of your organs like an amoeba might crawl across a petri dish.

These bloblike, voracious eaters are searching for any invaders that might have sneaked into your body. When an MP encounters one, it will capture it, cut it up into a thousand tiny pieces, and then take the bits and show them around the body to let the other troops, such as the B cells, know exactly what the invader looks like.

Sound overly dramatic? Actually, it's quite close to the literal truth. When macrophages encounter an invader, they grab it with amoebalike fingers and engulf it, swallowing the invader whole so that it becomes a captive. The macrophage then releases enzymes to digest it, breaking it down into tiny bits. These little sections become pieces of proteins—small enough to be moved around but large enough to provide a unique "fingerprint" identifying the invader the MP just gobbled up and digested.

The MP next spits up these little digested bits of protein fingerprints and displays them on its own surface, similar to placing a "Wanted" poster for the rest of your immune system to see. Now the B cells move in, going up to that "Wanted" poster, or that piece of the invader, and learning its shape. They then build an antibody that suits the shape of the invader perfectly. This antibody can now recognize and attach itself to the invader the next time it comes into contact with it.

The B cells next start making millions and millions of copies of this antibody, releasing them into the bloodstream. They float through our blood, and if they come into contact with one of these microbial invaders, the antibodies immediately attach themselves to it, triggering a series of events that will ultimately kill it.

Our B cells manufacture antibodies to exceptionally tight specifications so that the antibodies are specific to one particular germ. And the antibodies must be a perfect fit; otherwise, critical problems would result, the most important being that the antibody might not be properly able to recognize and neutralize the threat.

If, for instance, the antibody mistakenly grabbed onto your eye, you would go blind. If it grasped your brain, you'd suffer brain damage. As soon as antibodies take hold of something, a chain reaction is produced, and that thing will either be neutralized or killed.

Once a B cell learns to produce an antibody with the help of a macrophage, it retains the memory to produce that antibody forever. So in effect, that B cell is forever programmed to recognize a specific invader. If it ever encounters that invader again, the B cell will immediately begin producing millions of copies of its antibody, and will also reproduce itself thousands of times to create a force of so-called daughter cells. Each daughter cell also inherits the know-how to recognize that specific invader and to produce its specific antibody.

It is thought that B cells live anywhere from about a year to about six years. B cells reproduce themselves (by cell division) to maintain their collective memory, which is crucial for your very survival. And B cells can also multiply quickly in response to the recognition of a known threat. This ability to multiply helps build a formidable antibody response in the event a known invader gains entry into your body again.

There's a lot of brainpower in the B cells.

T CELLS

The other major group of lymphocytes is the T cells (T stands for thymus, the body organ in which they mature).

T cells look like B cells under a microscope—they are spherical, with a big nucleus and not much cytoplasm (the stuff that surrounds the nucleus). These T cells are the marines of your homeland security team. Just as every marine has a job classification, or a military occupational specialty (MOS), every T cell also has an MOS.

The T cells are divided into occupations such as helper T cells, suppressor T cells, and cytotoxic T cells. These are all very specialized functions, analogous to real marines assigned to the bomb squad, the recon team, and so forth. Some T cells (cytotoxic, or CD8, cells) attack invaders and infected cells directly, while others (helper, or CD4, cells and suppressor T cells) help regulate the immune response and keep it from becoming overactive. Cytotoxic (or cell-killing) T cells identify foreign organisms inside our cells and destroy those infected cells by recognizing changes in their surface proteins. They work in concert with the suppressor and helper T cells, which regulate the activity of the cytotoxic T cells.

Suppressor T cells help to regulate the immune reaction by preventing cytotoxic T cells from killing healthy cells. Helper, or CD4, T cells help cytotoxic cells kill infected cells. You may have heard of CD4 cells in the context of HIV infection, because these are the cells targeted by HIV (the human immunodeficiency virus). Low levels of CD4 cells signal a serious HIV infection.

Also important are specialized cells known as natural killer cells (NKs), which are assassins trained to destroy damaged, cancerous, or infected cells in the body. NK cells are similar to cytotoxic T cells but are more powerful.

Let's say you are exposed to a virus. One of the reasons viruses are so dangerous is that they don't just cruise around the tissue or blood and hide there, waiting for your body to destroy them. They actually creep inside your cells, and that means your body has to destroy some of its own cells if they become infected.

Once inside your cells, a virus messes with your DNA, tricking your cells into reproducing the virus by mingling its own DNA with yours. Then the virus uses your cells' DNA-processing system to replicate its own DNA too.

When a cell becomes infected with a virus in this way, the situation starts to resemble the scene from the science-fiction movie *Alien* in which the aliens, growing inside the characters' bodies, burst out, killing them.

Unfortunately, the only way to prevent the dangerous alien that is a virus from reproducing is to kill the newly infected cell. That's where the killer T cells come in. Natural killer cells sense a distress signal from the cells infected by a virus. The call may come from any type of cell—one that lines the nose or throat, or that resides in your intestines or in your skin.

When NK cells detect an infected cell, they use a special weapon to destroy it—a kind of plug that's injected into the cell membrane (the outside boundary of the cell). The plug, which has a small hole in it, is a protein called perforin. The NK cell then injects a substance called granzyme (or, more formally, exogenous serine protease) through the plug, which destroys the cell like a bomb.

That's how the natural killer cells work to destroy cells infected with viruses. Other parts of the immune system attack viruses directly, but natural killer T cells are those responsible for killing viral-infected cells, including the ones carrying HIV, which is why it's important to have a high count of NK cells in your blood.

Natural killer cells are involved in many search-and-destroy missions for our immune system. They're also important in killing cancerous cells that crop up in our bodies, ideally before they can grow into tumors. Cancer in the human body is not as rare as most people think; cancer cells are actually quite common. But for a number of reasons, most of these cells are never allowed to grow into tumors capable of killing us. One of the reasons for this is that the assassin-like NK cell snuffs them out before they have a chance to replicate.

Several therapies have been shown to increase NK activity, such as guided imagery, qigong, special breathing techniques, ginseng, and certain Chinese herbs.

HEMATOGENIC CELLS

Besides lymphocytes and macrophages, the third line of immune cells includes the blood-forming, or hematogenic, cells. Hematogenic cells are the cells from which our red blood cells, and many white blood cells, are produced. During a routine physical exam, your doctor probably performed a blood count, measuring the number and types of white blood cells seen in a drop of your blood. A high number (or high concentration) of white blood cells is usually a sign of some infection or stress on the body.

Many types of white blood cells are visible in a drop of blood. About half of them are known as neutrophils, aka polymorphonuclear cells, or polys for short.

I like calling these cells PMs, because that also stands for Pac-Man, the video game whose little creatures resemble PMs. Like Pac-Men, PMs sense invaders, chase after them, and once they've caught their quarry, they literally gobble them up.

Some of the other white blood cells include eosinophils, basophils, and monocytes. Each of these cells has its own specialized function. Eosinophils, for example, play a role in allergic reactions, as well as disorders like asthma. They are also involved in fighting off parasitic infestations.

As you know now, our immune system contains many specialized fighters possessing specialized weapons to deal with varied and sometimes uncommon threats. The ones mentioned above are just a few of the soldiers who are constantly fighting to keep your personal homeland safe. Right now, inside your body, they are all at work.

BORDER SECURITY AND THE ALTs

As discussed, one of the major duties of our body's homeland security system is border security, and it's a big border, including all of the surfaces that come into contact with the outside world. Invaders are constantly appearing, with the intent of not just looking around, but of doing us harm. Therefore, we need more than just a few cells of our immune system patrolling these borders.

This is where the so-called ALTs, or associated lymphoid tissues, enter the picture. ALTs are large clusters of immune cells located at fairly regular distances along our borders. For example, in the gut we have GALT (the gut-associated lymphoid tissue), which resembles thousands of strongholds positioned throughout the gut's lining, protecting the border between us and what's inside our gut.

The gut is an especially important border, not only because of its size (approximately the area of a tennis court when fully flattened), but also because of the constant barrage of bacteria and other microbes trying to break through it. The only barrier is a thin membrane a single cell thick.

Such a big assignment requires a large force, which is why the GALT alone accounts for about half of all the cells in our immune system. Most of these cells are T cells, but B cells, as well as macrophages, are also stationed in the GALT.

However, the borders of our homeland extend beyond the gut. There's also our skin, and the mucous membranes that line our nose, mouth, sinuses, throat, and lungs. Each of these boundaries needs its own defense force, so like the gut's GALT, we also have a SALT, a NALT, a TALT, and a BALT, whose acronyms stand for the skin-, nose-, throat- (or tonsils), and bronchial–associated lymphoid tissue. These aggregations of lymphoid tissue represent more than 70 percent of our immune system.

THE COMPLEMENT SYSTEM

We've already seen a number of ways our immune system's cells can fight off threats. For example, an MP (macrophage) or a PM (poly) can gobble up a germ, or an NK (natural killer) can inject a gran-zyme grenade into an infected cell.

There are several additional ways the immune system kills off bodily threats, using more sophisticated tools that allow it to rid the body of more than one invader at a time. After all, if faced with an invasion by billions of enemies, hand-to-hand combat alone won't work.

One of these tools is a chemical weapon known as an antibody, which is produced by the B cells. Yet another process occurs when the antibody nabs its target. The same handle, or tail, that signals to the immune system that it's caught something also triggers the deployment of a system of chemical weapons known as the comple-ment system.

The complement system is an exceedingly convoluted system of chemical warfare. In simple terms, think of the complement as something akin to an arsenal of nuclear weapons. The complement system is always present in our body, but its different components, of which there are at least thirty, are generally disassembled.

These complement components are produced mainly in the liver, but also by macrophages and other cells of the immune sys-tem. Separately, each of the complement components is harmless. But if the entire array is assembled, watch out! A nuclear reaction will take place.

The trigger for the complement construction transpires when those antibody pitchforks skewer so much prey it becomes clear additional help is needed. That critical level of battle initiates the assembly, or activation, of the complement system.

Activation of the complement system is one of the body's most impressive functions. Luckily, it is triggered only by severe issues, such as pneumococcal pneumonia or meningitis. It also occurs in organ transplantation—normally our immune system produces such a vigorous reaction to a transplanted organ that it causes organ rejection, which is why drugs must be given to suppress complement activation.

As in a nuclear reaction, once the complement system is activated, a process of events is triggered that is hard to stop and usually results in the death of the invaders.

That destruction takes the form of leaking capillaries, swelling, accumulation of lymph fluid, and the release of distress signals that attract even more fighters from all over the body, as well as the release of pyrogens (chemicals that raise body temperature, causing a fever) and general deployment of all available weapons, including nitric oxide and free radicals.

This entire process makes you feel very sick. If it continues, due to an overwhelming threat, it can lead to shock, organ failure, and death. Complement activation is therefore generally reserved for only the most serious circumstances.

THE COMMUNICATIONS SYSTEM

The final part of the homeland security detail you need to appreciate is the communications link.

For a battle in the outside world to go well, good communications are required: satellites, cell phones, radios, and microwave systems all communicate strategies as well as locate the enemy so it can be outflanked.

Your body has a similar kind of communications system.

The main category of communications devices is composed of the cytokines, of which more than one hundred have been discovered. Cytokines are proteins—such as interleukins, interferons, TNFs (tumor necrosis factors), pyrogens, and shock proteins—that send signals through your body to distant parts of the immune system.

Let's say you develop an ingrown toenail. First the Pac-Men engage with the enemy in the toe. But if they discover, say, an infection too powerful for them to fight on their own, they send out a message through the bloodstream that acts as both a distress and a homing signal, calling for reinforcements to the toe. This signal goes out in the form of cytokines.

Cytokines tell the rest of the immune cells where to go, and they follow the cytokines' scent just as a bloodhound sniffs out a trail, leading them right to the toe where the infection is wreaking havoc.

Drug companies are constantly researching cytokines and how to turn them on or off to treat different conditions. Cytokines are used to treat some infectious diseases, such as hepatitis, which is caused by a virus. For example, people are given interferon treatments if they are infected with hepatitis C. In autoimmune diseases such as rheumatoid arthritis or colitis, cytokine blockers including Enbrel, Humira, and Remicade are used to block the effects of the cytokines activating the immune system.

The immune system is so complicated that it would take volumes to explain all its details. But this brief introduction should provide you with a basic understanding. Knowing how your immune system operates can save your life—the more you know about it, the better you will treat it, and, in return, the better it will treat you.

HOW THE IMMUNE SYSTEM
CAN GO WRONG

THE IMMUNE SYSTEM is remarkable for its size, complexity, and efficiency. But like the human beings in whom it resides, the immune system can be quite fallible. The weakness lies primarily in two areas: on the one hand, the potential to be overpowered by invaders, and on the other, overstimulation.

The first problem occurs when our immune system musters an inadequate response to foreign invaders, who then pass through the defense network. We know this process all too well—an infection takes hold and our immune system isn't capable of fighting it. This might happen when a particularly nasty infection flares from a killer germ, causing, for example, typhoid, diphtheria, or tetanus.

Another possibility is that the immune system itself has been rendered almost powerless by some invader (such as HIV), by certain conditions (such as immunodeficiency diseases), or by an immune-suppressing medication (such as antirejection drugs taken by transplant recipients, or, more commonly, steroids such as prednisone or cortisone). In such cases, our immune system can't defend us from the invaders that it would otherwise easily dispose of.

Unfortunately, failure of the immune system remains the primary killer in developing nations, which have historically lacked access to modern vaccines and antibiotics, as well as to proper sanitation, clean water, and healthy food. (In fact, in developing countries millions die every year simply from contaminated water.) Diseases such as tuberculosis, malaria, and cholera are still among the world's biggest killers.

In a way, the type of aging process discussed in this book is specifically a disease of people in affluent, developed nations. In Nigeria, there are few nursing homes for Alzheimer's patients. In the Sudan, few bypass surgeries are performed. Only a small number of significant problems from the diseases of aging exist in the developing world, because people often don't live long enough to experience them.

In other words, in third world countries, the immune system struggles just to do its job against the vast array of invaders still prevalent in the landscape. The situation is different in the developed world. Rather than infectious diseases, more than 50 percent of American deaths in 2005 were due to autoimmune problems, while only 4 percent were caused directly by infection (flu, pneumonia, sepsis). The remainder of American deaths include about 6 percent caused by injury (accidents, suicide) and 23 percent by cancer (aided and abetted by the immune system, as we'll discuss later).

In America, we have the luxury of the technological and economic advantages that prolong life and, in part, contribute to the development of an aging population and the attendant diseases of aging.

This is not a bad thing, nor something about which we should feel guilty. After all, we are in a position to conduct the best research on aging and the immune system. Once medicine and public health measures are able to rid the external environment of the sources of attacks on our health, we may find a cure for the diseases of aging too—saving developing nations from having to reinvent the wheel in regard to bolstering the immune system.

IMMUNE ACTIVATION: THE CRP TEST

In our environment, the more dangerous peril occurs when the immune system becomes overactive.

The first research group to study and recognize the association between immune activation and conditions such as heart disease, stroke, and poor circulation was led by Dr. Paul Ridker, of Harvard Medical School, in the mid-1990s. While conducting research on the heart, Ridker noticed high levels of C-reactive protein (CRP) in the blood of patients who had had heart attacks.

The most common test for immune system activation is a CRP blood test—the higher the CRP level, the more active the immune system. (Another common way to measure immune system activity is sedimentation, or sed, rate. Sed rate measures how fast red blood cells settle to the bottom of a test tube of blood; the faster they settle, the more active the immune system, because when the immune system is active, the blood contains more proteins, such as CRP and other cytokines that adhere to red blood cells and make them stick together. That causes the red blood cells to fall, or "sediment," more quickly, raising the sed rate.)

Repeated studies by Ridker's group showed that CRP levels were also a better predictor of heart attack than cholesterol, blood pressure, family history, or any other of the traditional risk factors.

Although a basic CRP test had been available for several years before Ridker's research, his group was instrumental in developing a far more sensitive test able to detect CRP levels to a much greater degree of accuracy.

Development of this highly sensitive CRP test (hs-CRP) was a key step in identifying the link between immune activation and heart disease, because Ridker found that even slightly elevated levels of CRP increased the heart attack risk. The hs-CRP test was more accurate than any other test in medical history at helping the researchers distinguish between people who were likely to be safe from heart attack and those who were at risk.

Many other researchers have since confirmed Ridker's findings. What's even more interesting is that elevations of hs-CRP have now been found to predict many other diseases besides heart disease. Elevated hs-CRP has been found to be an excellent predictor of the following: abdominal aortic aneurysms, Alzheimer's disease, atrial fibrillation (irregular heartbeat), diabetes, high blood pressure, macular degeneration (a leading cause of blindness), osteoporosis, stroke, sudden cardiac death, and colon, prostate, and other cancers.

Note that CRP levels become elevated even before the diseases themselves are present, meaning that immune activation precedes the diseases.

Scientists are just beginning to understand and identify the specific involvement of the immune system in actually *causing* these diseases. What medical researchers have come to realize, thanks in part to the pioneering work of people like Dr. Ridker, is that friendly fire can take place just as easily inside a body as outside it.

Medically speaking, what is friendly fire? In a real war, innocent bystanders can be hurt. The same is true inside your body. If your immune system is waging a battle to defend you from a threat, its ammunition may accidentally harm innocent bystanders—your heart, brain, blood vessels, pancreas, or any other guiltless spectator that the immune system isn't trying to destroy, but that may nonetheless become injured by friendly fire.

In the process of protecting us, the immune system aims to target a specific infection, but it is not able to coordinate its forces so precisely that only the infection itself is attacked. When its many weapons hit other parts of the body, it can create serious problems.

It's easy to see why the balance between protection and destruction in our immune system is critical, because when it is out of whack, illnesses can result.

CYNTHIA'S STORY

Cynthia first came to see me because she had been diagnosed with uveitis, a disease of the middle layers of the eye that often leads to blindness; in fact, uveitis is the fifth leading cause of blindness in the United States. Needless to say, Cynthia was concerned, especially because no one could tell her what was causing her condition.

Cynthia said that her ophthalmologist was monitoring her closely, that she saw him every four months, and that he'd prescribed daily steroid drops to keep her immune system from damaging her eyesight. But the drops worried Cynthia; she knew they could cause serious side effects, such as cataracts. Still, her doctor informed her that her choice was either blindness from uveitis or cataracts, which could be removed.

Cynthia, fit and active, was otherwise healthy—but she did suffer from heartburn. And when we tested her CRP, we found it elevated—3.3 milligrams per liter, or about five times higher than ideal. Cynthia's immune system was obviously highly activated. We immediately wondered if the bacterium involved might be *Helicobacter pylori*, which not only activates the immune system but can cause heartburn. Because a simple blood test to screen for *Helicobacter* is available, we immediately tested Cynthia. She proved positive.

The treatment for this infection is a two-week course of combination antibiotics, one of the only proven ways to eradicate this specific bacterium. Three months after she took the treatment, Cynthia's eye doctor could find no evidence of uveitis. Cynthia told us that the doctor was guardedly optimistic but remained unconvinced of a link between uveitis and *Helicobacter*.

At a follow-up appointment two months later, however, there was still no evidence of uveitis. Amazed, the doctor asked to see Cynthia in two more months; once again, no uveitis. Cynthia's ophthalmologist then began testing all of his uveitis patients for *Helicobacter* infection.

Two years later, in the journal *Infection* (April 1, 2005), came the first report in the medical literature confirming the link between H. *pylori* infection and uveitis. What the researchers had found was that antibodies to H. *pylori* had somehow ended up inside the eyes of patients with uveitis.

Cynthia's case is a perfect example of friendly fire. In trying to fight and eradicate an infection in the stomach, her B cells reproduced and manufactured antibodies against it. These antibodies traveled through the bloodstream in search of their intended target, but as sometimes happens, they missed it and injured innocent bystanders instead. Rather than attack their intended target, *Helicobacter*, the antibodies found their way into Cynthia's eyes and triggered an immune reaction that could have eventually caused blindness.

THE LINK BETWEEN AGING AND AN OVERACTIVE IMMUNE SYSTEM

The older you are, the more likely a debacle such as Cynthia's is to occur. This is due, in part, to the enormous database of different invaders your immune system has built over time.

Because of this memory, the immune system reacts with growing force to an increasing number of foreigners it has identified. Eventually, your body may build up such a large storehouse of data that your immune system becomes confused as to what's part of you and what isn't.

Studies show that as we age, more and more organ-specific antibodies are found in our bloodstream. As the name suggests, organ-specific antibodies are produced by our immune system (B cells and their daughters) to attack specific organs themselves, such as the pancreas, brain, and liver. A study from Palermo, Italy, for example (published in *Mechanisms of Aging and Development*, March 1997), compared the levels of organ-specific antibodies in young, old, and very old individuals. The finding: numbers of antibodies increased with age. The one exception concerned people living to be older than one hundred years. Among these centenarians, there was no increase in the number of organ-specific antibodies compared with young people. One of the important features of living to be a hundred or older is having an absence of organ-specific antibodies.

Why would our immune system produce antibodies against our own organs? As we get older, the number of memories in our immune system's database multiplies because it is constantly being exposed to new and different things. It's unavoidable that some of the antibodies produced in response to viruses or foods, for example, turn out to cross-react with our own organs. As the database grows, so does the chance that some of these antibodies will attack our own tissue, not just the virus or bacteria that were being targeted. But for those healthy centenarians who have benefited from a healthy immune system that is not overreacting, there is an absence of organ-specific antibodies.

This and similar studies suggest that a major factor in aging well is the absence of organ-specific antibodies. In other words, the quieter your immune system, the healthier you are—which is exactly what the Seven-Step UltraLongevity Program will help you achieve.

THE IMMUNE SYSTEM AND INVADERS

Just as our country's defense system would be sorely tested if several invaders attacked simultaneously, so, too, when your body has to deal with many potential terrorists, the opportunities for breakdowns multiply.

This confusion leads to malfunction of the immune system, and that malfunction leads to bodily damage.

The process through which immune activation damages our body has come to be understood via research on several conditions, particularly atherosclerosis, or the hardening of the arteries that leads to heart attack, stroke, and other circulatory crises.

Atherosclerosis is caused by a buildup of plaque in the walls of the arteries. This buildup can occur in any artery, from the carotid arteries in the neck to those in the aorta or in the brain. Many different kinds of plaque exist, but the kind that builds up inside your arteries is composed of fat (lipid) that is mostly cholesterol, along with a mix of cells (e.g., macrophages and fibroblasts) and a chemical soup whose ingredients include cytokines, enzymes, and free radicals.

Plaque accumulates slowly in people with high cholesterol, high blood pressure, certain genetic factors, and/or who smoke. Plaque buildup becomes dangerous and can lead to a heart attack or stroke at the point when the immune system becomes activated. This scenario commonly occurs as follows.

For any one of many different reasons, such as in response to an infection, stress, sleep deprivation, or low oxygen, a signal is sent out as a generalized call to arms for the immune system. As discussed earlier, this signal is sent by cytokines, released by our white blood cells.

At the cytokines' bugle call, the macrophages (MPs) are activated and, like a bloodhound tracking a scent, they sniff around for possible invaders or hot spots of engagement with the enemy. MPs then stick to the lining of the blood vessels and, once they grab hold, start to burrow into the wall of the artery itself in search of their prey.

Once inside the artery wall, the MPs gobble up anything that looks like it doesn't belong, such as small cholesterol particles that have accumulated. Assuming they are fighting an enemy, MPs then release more cytokines, which magnify the immune activation at that spot. Still more macrophages are called in, which follow the cytokines' "scent" to the same spot.

Other cells, such as T and dendritic cells, also follow the chemical signals until a small, microscopic battle is being fought inside the artery wall.

Each of these fighters releases its own chemical weapons, from antibodies to free radicals to enzymes that digest proteins, and soon enough the tiny battleground becomes like a boil in the artery wall—a juicy plaque that can rupture and burst into the artery. This rupture then causes a blood clot to form that blocks off blood flow to the artery, which in turn can prompt a heart attack, a stroke, or some other circulatory disaster.

Similarly, in brain diseases such as Alzheimer's, damage to nerve cells in the brain also stems from immune activation. The original activation, or call to arms, may have begun for some entirely unrelated reason, at a site very distant from the brain. It could originate in an infection, or be due to obesity, a lack of physical fitness, or hundreds of other microbattles being fought in arterial plaques throughout the body.

In the brain, MPs are called microglial cells, or microglia. These MPs in the brain are activated by the same signals—cytokines, CRP, and so on—and start gobbling up anything that doesn't seem to belong. Often these foreign-seeming targets are deposits of a protein called amyloid. Once an MP gobbles up foreign protein like amyloid, it triggers a chain reaction that leads, once again, to an overzealous immune response. Such an overactive response in the brain damages neurons and ultimately causes the loss of brain function characteristic of Alzheimer's disease.

Other conditions characterized by an overactive immune response include arthritis, diabetes, osteoporosis, asthma, stroke, high blood pressure, emphysema, and obesity.

LEONARD'S STORY

I first met seventy-nine-year-old Lennie in October of 2003; he was referred by his brother, whom I had been treating for many years.

Lennie was having a serious problem: progressive atherosclerosis and an impending heart attack. After suffering chest pains, followed by breathing difficulties, he saw his doctor, who correctly recommended immediate hospitalization and cardiac testing. What scared Lennie was that his doctor told him he would probably need a bypass. As this was the last thing he wanted to hear, and feeling that he was old enough to simply refuse and seek out other options, he asked his brother for help.

After our first consultation, I felt that Lennie's immune system

---

AGING SPURTS

When people think of getting older, they think in terms of time, as if we age as the hands on the clock move—a second, a minute, an hour, a day older. Actually, the passing of time and the aging of humans aren't equivalent. Aging takes place in spurts.

We're all familiar with growth spurts. If you have children, you've noticed their growth rate is variable. Some weeks they seem to grow a full inch, while at other times they don't seem to develop at all.

It's recently been discovered that we age in a similar way. Remember that aging takes place as our cells die. Of course, that's very different from human growth and development. Children are not *aging* as they grow into adults; they are *maturing* into the full expression of life. Aging, in contrast, is a process of senescence, or of loss of function that stems from the loss of cells and organ reserve—which comes about from an overactive immune system. The process of aging doesn't even begin until we've fully matured into our late twenties or early thirties.

---

was probably overactivated—chest pains and shortness of breath would get anyone's system riled up. But Lennie was also experiencing aches all over his body—which he attributed to age—and he felt tired, mentally sluggish, and had gained a little weight.

A quick blood test confirmed our suspicions. Lennie's CRP level was a whopping 15.8 (ideally, it should be less than 0.7). There were other abnormalities. Lennie's blood sugar was high, suggesting a trend toward diabetes. His blood pressure was also elevated, and his white blood cell count was higher than ideal. Lennie was showing all the classic signs of immune hyperactivity.

The real question was not what was wrong, but was it too late?

Of course we all were nervous about the possibility that Lennie's immune system had been allowed to remain on high for too

---

But like growth, aging happens in spurts. These are periods during which we lose organ function much more quickly than at other times. The impact of these spurts depends on the degree to which our immune system is overactivated; the more intense and prolonged the activation, the more profound the aging spurt.

How many times have you looked at someone and thought that he or she had grown much older in only a short time? If you looked under his or her hood, so to speak, you'd find all kinds of evidence of immune activation: high CRP levels, high white blood cell counts, and activated white blood cells patrolling the body in the search-and-destroy mode.

On the other hand, when you see someone who looks much younger than his or her age, he or she usually seems calm, peaceful, healthy, and seldom overeats. Inside you'd be likely to find low CRP levels, low white blood cell counts, low interleukin levels, and so on.

In order to slow down the aging process, you need to avoid aging spurts caused by unnecessary immune activation. By so doing, you will be able to live an extraordinarily long and healthy life.

---

long. But Lennie was quite adamant—he did not want a bypass, angiogram, or stent.

We immediately started him on our UltraLongevity program to bring his immune system under control. The program began with breathing exercises in the form of qigong and tai chi, as well as a daily walking program. Lennie's new diet now consisted of low-calorie meals that were high in fiber and low in sugar. To accompany his diet, he started taking supplements with the B vitamins, vitamins C and E, and fish oil, along with aspirin and Lipitor, a cholesterol-lowering statin drug that can have a beneficial effect on immune activation.

To soothe the man, his soul, and his immune system, we also made sure that Lennie took massages and surrounded himself with calming aromas and music.

Lennie followed the program to the letter. Within just two weeks he was feeling much better. After seven weeks, his CRP level had dropped from 15.8 to 1.4, his blood sugar had normalized, he had lost eleven pounds, and his blood pressure had dropped twenty points.

Lennie enthusiastically continued the program. Eight weeks later, his CRP was down to 0.4. Lennie felt great and had no further symptoms. There was no longer any sign of immune activation; he had successfully bypassed the bypass. Lennie continues to do well and remains on the program.

As discussed earlier, our immune system, much like the country's Department of Homeland Security, has two main tasks:

1. To respond to disasters and emergencies
2. To provide border security

As you will learn, when these jobs are not being handled correctly, immune overactivation—and therefore aging—results.

DISASTERS AND EMERGENCY RESPONSES

Responding to disasters and emergencies is a surefire way for our immune system to become overly activated.

PHYSICAL INJURY

Physical injury is one type of disaster. Say you break your leg. You suffer a stab wound. You're shot. The immune reaction to that kind of injury is extremely intense. (In homeland security terms, these crises are the equivalent of a hurricane, volcanic eruption, or a bombing.)

When someone with a serious injury enters a hospital emergency room, his or her immune system is out of control. It's easy to measure: the white blood count is sky-high, the sed rate is off the map, the CRP level is through the roof. The immune system is responding in the most overwhelming way it can to devastating injury, flooding white blood cells into the bloodstream and to the site of the injury itself.

For example, if the injury is a stab wound, the immune system has to defend against that wound by sealing off the hole, killing the bacteria that went through it, and figuring out what happened—it can't understand what took place until its scouts arrive and assess the damage. At first, all the immune system knows is that the body has set off an alarm due to a disaster. Because the trauma could be lethal, the immune system has to assume, and act, as though it's something that could quickly kill.

Thus, injuries are one form of bodily emergency that produces a powerful reaction by your immune system.

Often, when I ask my patients how an elderly relative passed away, I hear, "She died of a hip fracture." The truth is that no one really dies of the hip fracture itself. It hurts, of course, but there aren't any vital structures in the hip whose injury would be lethal. Yet according to a study in *JAMA* (June 6, 2001), the mortality rate from hip fractures is 13.5 percent in the first six months after the injury for patients over fifty.

These deaths are due to the immune activation that occurs as a result of the injury. This immune activation leads to higher rates of heart attacks, strokes, and lethal blood clots—and these are what can kill.

HYPOXIA

Another type of emergency is hypoxia, or low oxygen. Hypoxia occurs in situations such as drowning, asphyxiation, being in high altitudes, and in sleep apnea, a common condition in which people stop breathing while sleeping because their airway gets blocked when their tongue slips to the back of their throat (*apnea* is Greek for "no breathing"). Because the person is asleep, he or she can't respond. The oxygen level starts to drop, and once it gets too low, the person is usually aroused and wakes up just long enough to resume breathing.

Repeated tests show that people with sleep apnea have very high CRP levels. And when the sleep apnea is corrected, those levels drop—evidence that the immune system is activated whenever hypoxia occurs.

Impaired lung function has also been linked with immune activation, because it usually causes hypoxia. In a review of fourteen published studies (reported in *Thorax*, 2004), reduced lung function was found to be associated with evidence of immune activation, including elevated CRP, elevated white blood cell count, and the presence of cytokines such as tumor necrosis factor alpha (TNF-alpha).

You can live only three to four minutes without oxygen. But even if you survive, oxygen deprivation causes a great deal of damage to the body, and is a loud and clear signal to the immune system that you are in grave danger.

INFECTIONS AND OTHER ATTACKS

A third type of emergency is the equivalent of a terrorist attack on your homeland soil. The culprits can be any of hundreds of evildoers, including strep bacteria, avian flu, pneumonia, kidney infection, or bronchitis.

All of these terrorists have the potential to kill you. Thus they, too, cause a vigorous immune system activation. In fact, medical science has found that the greater the number of serious infections people have suffered, the greater their risk of conditions such as heart attack, stroke, and cancer.

In a study reported in the *American Journal of Cardiology* in 2003, researchers found a strong association between the number of antibodies to specific microbes (e.g., *Chlamydia pneumonia*, cytomegalovirus, herpes simplex virus 1, and *Helicobacter pylori*) and the presence of coronary artery disease (blockages and narrowing in the arteries supplying the heart). In other words, the more frequently a person has been infected, the more likely he or she is to have coronary artery disease.

Supported by funding from the National Institute on Aging, Eileen Crimmins and Caleb Finch of the University of Southern California School of Gerontology studied eighteenth- and nineteenth-century European public health records. Their research showed that generations of people who had survived rampant childhood infections lived shorter lives than those generations who suffered fewer childhood diseases. The authors suggested that battling repeated childhood infections caused immune activation, which increased the likelihood of dying from cardiovascular disease at a relatively young age later in life.

Infection has also been linked with cancer. Renowned Greek physician Galen first noted the connection between the two almost two thousand years ago. Since then, many infections have been linked with several different types of cancer. Currently, infections by bacteria and viruses account for one-fifth of cancers worldwide.

Some of the infections linked to cancer include the already mentioned *Helicobacter pylori* (stomach cancer), schistosomiasis (bladder cancer), Epstein-Barr virus (lymphoma), human papillomavirus (cervical cancer), and hepatitis B and C (liver cancer).

Chronic infections of any kind seem to increase the risk of cancer. For example, chronic bone infection (osteomyelitis) is known to cause bone cancer, and chronic bronchitis has been linked with lung cancer. In February 2006, researchers at the University of California in San Francisco found a virus in human prostate tumors never before detected, suggesting a possible link between viral infections and prostate cancer.

Chronic infections have also been linked with brain diseases, such as dementia and Alzheimer's disease. In 1998, researchers at the Hahnemann School of Medicine in Philadelphia identified the presence of a bacterium called *Chlamydia pneumoniae* in the brains of seventeen of nineteen Alzheimer's disease patients tested.

In fact, brain changes characteristic of Alzheimer's disease can be produced in mice simply by giving them a sinus infection with the same *Chlamydia* bacteria (*Neurobiology of Aging*, April 2004). Other infections, such as herpes, have also been linked with Alzheimer's (*Neurobiology of Aging*, May–June 2004).

Infections have also been implicated in many of the classic autoimmune disorders. For example, strep throat infections are known to trigger autoimmune kidney disease and valvular heart disease. Strep throat itself is not terribly frightening; almost everyone can recover on their own. But if the strep is not treated with antibiotics, people are much more likely to develop autoimmune kidney disease and heart valve problems (rheumatic heart disease). Before the discovery of penicillin in the late 1920s, the rates of rheumatic fever and rheumatic heart disease were sky-high compared with today's rates.

Infections have also been implicated as a cause of multiple sclerosis (human herpesvirus), rheumatoid arthritis (strep infections), Crohn's disease (*Mycobacterium paratuberculosis*), myocarditis (coxsackie B virus), and other autoimmune diseases.

As all of this information makes clear, our immune system's immediate reaction to a specific infection causes a lasting activation that continues long after the initial infection has been eradicated—causing problems than can last a lifetime.

CANCER

Cancer can be considered out-and-out war in your body. The immune system becomes highly activated anytime cancer is growing, and the potential for damage is enormous.

A great deal of evidence now suggests that our body is fighting cancer skirmishes all the time. Not infrequently, one of the cells somewhere in our body has a DNA mutation that transforms it into a cancer cell. These DNA mutations occur for any number of reasons, including exposure to radiation, a toxic-level exposure to some chemical, or as a by-product of our own metabolism—from a virus infecting the cell, free radical damage inside a cell, or simply one of the errors that sometimes occur during cell division and reproduction.

When detailed autopsies are conducted, researchers often find cancerous cells, even though the person in question didn't die of cancer. For example, up to a third of autopsies show microscopic cancer in the thyroid gland, and more than 80 percent of men eighty years or older have cancerous prostate cells at autopsy.

Although cancer frequently arises on a cellular basis, these cancerous cells don't usually grow into lethal tumors, because our immune system detects and kills the abnormal cells early. Our immune system is constantly patrolling for cells that might be cancerous. Detecting them, however, can be a tricky business because of the cells' nature.

Cancer cells begin as normal cells, but due to mutation, they lose control of the natural process that regulates their division and reproduction. Soon, cancer cells begin dividing and multiplying very rapidly—one cell becomes two cells, two become four, four become eight, and so on, until a potentially lethal tumor with millions of cells has formed.

The problem here is that our immune system perceives these cancer cells as part of us; unless the mutation causes a bizarre cell to develop, cancer cells can be very difficult for our immune system to distinguish from our own normal cells. This creates a serious challenge. The similarity between cancerous cells and our own normal cells creates a kind of cloaking mechanism that enables the former to go undetected by the immune system, which then allows these cells to grow unchecked into tumors.

One other step has to take place before a cancer cell will turn into a tumor: a separate blood supply must be created. Tumors are solid masses of cells, and every cell needs nourishment—even a cancer cell. The potential tumor requires the same fuels for growth as the rest of our cells—protein, sugar, vitamins, and minerals. In fact, because of cancer cells' rapid growth, a tumor often needs more blood flow than a collection of normal cells.

Tumors develop their own blood supply through a process called angiogenesis. *Angio* means "blood vessel," and *genesis* means "beginning," so angiogenesis means the beginning or initiation of blood vessels. What's surprising is that our own immune system may unknowingly contribute to the process of angiogenesis by producing compounds known as angiogenic growth factors. In the case of a growing cancerous tumor, extra blood flow is not good. Unfortunately, our immune system can unwittingly contribute. Here's why this process develops:

Most likely, macrophages on patrol identify a growing tumor, which they recognize as foreign and a likely threat. Therefore, they attack. The MPs start fighting the tumor the same way they would fight any other threat—by gobbling up some tumor cells, releasing cytokines, and calling in more MPs and other fighting cells for help.

In their effort to protect you, the MPs also start triggering more blood flow. The intention is to bring more blood to the area to help with their defensive actions. If fighting an infection, that's a good thing. More blood flow means more circulation, which helps fight an infection by diluting and washing away the germs or bacteria responsible. In the case of cancer, however, additional blood flow to the tumor has the opposite effect, bringing more nutrients into the tumor, fueling its growth.

More blood flow may also have the dire consequence of helping cancerous cells break off from the main tumor and spread to distant locations in the body. This process, known as metastasis, is the way cancer eventually becomes lethal. Growing and spreading cancer is deadly, and in this way our immune system becomes an unwitting accomplice in the process. It is another form of friendly fire.

We are just beginning to learn how to control our immune system in ways that instruct it to kill the cancerous cells, and not to aid and abet their growth unintentionally. The strategy of blocking the tumor-feeding effects so that tumors can't grow is called anti-angiogenesis therapy. Pharmaceutical companies are spending billions of dollars every year in a race to develop the first blockbuster anti-angiogenesis drugs.

What's exciting is that many different compounds have been shown to block blood vessel growth into tumors, some of which are vitamins, herbs, and food extracts in addition to prescription and nonprescription medications. The possibility of using a number of readily available and fairly nontoxic compounds to curtail the growth and spread of cancer is a hopeful new discovery that allows us to harness the power of our immune system while blocking its negative actions.

GENES AND IMMUNITY

One of the questions I hear most often is, "How do my genes affect immunity and aging?" The answer is: We don't really know.

Medical researchers have identified dozens of genes that seem to regulate immune system function; examples include the genes that encode for the production of antibodies and those responsible for producing cytokines. Medical science is also identifying certain genes affecting the immune system and longevity that vary slightly from person to person. These genetic differences may help explain the variation in immune function and the speed of aging among individuals.

But for better or worse, we are all born with a set of genes that we possess our entire lives. Of course, our genes come from our parents, so most of us have an idea of what might be in store. But the shuffling and mixing of our parents' genes means we won't follow our parents' genetic path step for step.

As genetic testing becomes more commonplace, we're discovering more about the specific genes we all carry. The Human Genome Project has now mapped the entire human genome— identifying each and every gene humans possess. Yet that project

EMOTIONS

Another area of immune system activation is in response to perceived but unverifiable disasters. Our immune system possesses numerous strategies for monitoring our bodily homeland for possible threats, including tapping into our emotions. That's right: our immune system monitors our emotions to gain an early advantage.

This ability has evolved over eons to insure our survival. Our immune system is smart enough to realize the importance of knowing that we are, for example, afraid; fear is often followed by pain, infection, injury, and even death. The immune system perceives identified only the thirty thousand common human genes rather than the slight genetic variations we all carry, and it's these slight variations that make each of us unique.

For those of you who take a proactive approach to your health, knowing your genetic makeup may help you to better direct your preventive efforts. For example, if your genes indicate an increased risk for heart disease, controlling cholesterol and blood pressure may be more important for you than for someone who's not at risk.

However, because the immune system is so pivotal in the process of disease and aging, everyone should be trying to improve it, regardless of genetic history.

The bottom line is that, as far as we now know, genetic testing can tell us only about future risks, possibilities, and probabilities. It can't tell us what our immune system is doing right now. It can't tell us whether it is reacting to our emotional state or to an infection, for example. It can't tell us about the ongoing effects of our environment, our feelings, our habits, or our stresses. So no matter how good genetic testing becomes, it probably won't provide the final answer to explain or improve the state of our health. Despite our genes, our immune system will remain a key factor controlling our health and the speed of aging.

fear as a threat, or at least a warning of a possible one. Similarly, the immune system recognizes hostility, despair, and frustration as possible dangers.

New medical research shows that when we are afraid, angry, or depressed, we are more likely to contract the diseases linked with aging. In a ten-year study of young adults published in JAMA (May 17, 2000), the degree of hostility measured was correlated with a buildup of calcified plaque in the coronary arteries. In this same study, hostility was also linked with the development of high blood pressure; the greater the hostility felt, the higher the risk of high blood pressure.

A study from Duke University's Behavioral Sciences Department, published in *Psychosomatic Medicine* in September/October 2004, found that a higher degree of anger and hostility predicted higher CRP levels.

Anxiety, too, has been shown to activate the immune system; in a 2004 study of 1,100 men and women, the degree of fear of a terrorist attack one experienced was correlated with the level of immune activation (*Psychosomatic Medicine*, July/August 2004).

Depression and despair also have immune-activating effects. As reported in *Biological Psychiatry* (April 7, 2006), in a Finnish study of more than five thousand people, the presence of severe depression in men was linked with elevated CRP. Depression was linked with higher CRP levels in a study of 127 men and women, published in *Psychosomatic Medicine* (September/October 2004).

For some time, medical science has suspected a powerful connection between emotions and health, but only now are we beginning to understand why this connection exists and how it works. Research shows that a key to preventing heart disease lies in the ability to manage emotions. This is why biofeedback, meditation, yoga, compassionate thinking, and other means of working with one's emotions can, and do, nullify or mitigate the adverse effects of fear, hostility, and depression.

How, then, does our immune system sense these emotions? Very much the same way our brain would, it turns out: via chemical messengers, including adrenaline, serotonin, dopamine, and other neurotransmitters.

Scientists still don't know where in the body emotions originate. Most likely, they start in the brain, along with thoughts, but this is still only a theory—other hypotheses place the seat of emotions in the nerve centers in the gut.

What is known is that certain chemicals are released into our bloodstream when we experience specific emotions. Fear, for example, causes the release of adrenaline, cortisol, and a blend of other chemicals. Love seems to be linked with a mix of dopamine and oxytocin. The exact pattern and chemical fingerprint of each emotion has not been entirely deciphered—feelings are complex things.

What is clear is that it's not just the brain that creates or senses emotional states. Research has shown that the immune system is also very involved.

In her book *Molecules of Emotion*, National Institute of Health researcher Candace Pert describes how she was able to prove that white blood cells of the immune system contain receptors that sense the same neurotransmitters the brain uses to communicate emotions, such as adrenaline, serotonin, oxytocin, and dopamine. In other words, our immune system has a well-developed procedure to sense our emotions and then respond to the threat that caused them.

JENNIFER'S STORY

Fifty-two-year-old Jennifer was stuck. Suffering from high blood pressure, elevated cholesterol, and fatigue, she was also extremely depressed, caused primarily by one factor: her husband had developed full-blown Alzheimer's disease.

Whenever Jennifer came in for checkups, we would spend most of our time talking about her coping strategies. But despite our best efforts, we couldn't find a way to free Jennifer from the grip of depression.

At each checkup, her CRP and white blood count were elevated. Despite a regular exercise program, a healthy diet, and medication for blood pressure and cholesterol, Jennifer's immune system remained on full alert.

Not unexpectedly, Jennifer's husband passed away. Jennifer honored the grieving process and worked with a therapist to understand what had happened and where she now stood in life. After a long absence, she returned to Canyon Ranch. Again we noted that her symptoms were still present, and above all, that her CRP levels remained high.

We asked her to start the UltraLongevity program. Because each patient has different needs, not everyone pays the same degree of attention to each step. In Jennifer's case, she needed to work on her emotions. We prescribed daily walks, yoga, and qigong breathing exercises. She also continued the work of grieving and added a therapy known as Eye Movement Desensitization and Reprocessing. This new therapy helped Jennifer deal with the trauma of loss and with post-traumatic stress disorder.

The program slowly began to work. Jennifer reported back that she was feeling better.

I didn't see her in person for another six months. The entire staff was startled, and pleased, when she returned. After working diligently on improving her mood and supporting her immune system, Jennifer had undergone a complete transformation. Her affect was lighter, her appearance more youthful, and she had lost thirty pounds. She had tried every diet under the sun until now, but by working specifically on supporting her immune system, she had finally found a way to lose the weight. Furthermore, her blood pressure was the lowest we had ever measured, and so was her cholesterol. And her immune system markers were now into the optimal range.

Jennifer reported that she couldn't remember ever feeling better. She was energetic, spry, and had a positive attitude about her life. Her health had been restored.

BORDER SECURITY

Our immune system must patrol the body's borders—the areas where our body ends and the outside world begins. This border is huge, and includes not just our skin and our respiratory tract, but our reproductive tract and gut as well. (Think about the gut for a moment. Humans ingest a great deal of food; the immune system must investigate all of it to find potentially dangerous hitchhikers.)

The possible entry points for invaders cover an enormous area, all of which the immune system must study—as mentioned, the surface area of the small intestine alone is the size of a tennis court. If you add the surface area of the lungs, about eight hundred square feet, and the skin, about twenty square feet, you'll realize that your immune system is continuously patrolling a border about 80 percent as large as a professional basketball court.

Our border patrol protects us ably, but it can also be a cause of an overactive immune system and thus prematurely age us. For example, consider people who have been exposed to strep bacteria. The tonsils react to the bacteria, which activates a visible immune response not only in the throat itself, but also in the entire immune system. Why? The immune response to strep is so powerful that it provokes a massive mobilization of antibodies and activation of the complement system. This level of overwhelming response can clog up the kidneys with antibodies, complement, and cytokines, and can even trigger kidney failure.

Overactive border patrol in the lungs is the cause of asthma— immune cells there responding to inhaled threats such as pollens, dust, or smoke can trigger a reaction that produces a swelling and constriction of the airways, which in turn leads to shortness of breath, coughing, and wheezing—asthma. In other words, it's the immune system's overreaction that causes someone to breathe poorly, not the inhalant itself.

FRIEND VS. FOES

Not every alien that makes it over the border will trigger an immune response, and rightly so. Over millions of years our immune system has evolved to be able to recognize the difference between friendly tourists and hostile terrorists.

Friendly tourists enter our body because they are either idly passing through us or intend to stay and befriend us (rather than to launch an attack). Most of the microbes living around and within our bodies mean us no harm, including the microscopic mites that inhabit our eyebrows and the friendly bacteria that live on our skin. In fact, some of these foreigners are more than just tourists—they are essential parts of our system. You could say that our immune system subcontracts with other security forces to help out in the process of protecting us.

In the gut, for example, our immune system employs symbiotic bacteria to help us defend our health. "Symbiotic" means that these bacteria and our bodies mutually assist each other. It's a sort of food-for-hire program in which the bacteria make a living wage of feasting on the indigestible portion of our diets in return for helping to protect the gut's border from nastier potential terrorist bacteria, yeasts, and hostile microbes.

Successfully subcontracting some of the security duties to healthy, desirable bacteria is an important strategy for preventing autoimmune diseases, immune activation, and aging. Scientific evidence is mounting that our immune system absolutely needs these types of organisms in order to mature and function properly.

ANTIBIOTICS: A DOUBLE-EDGED SWORD

One of the problems associated with frequent antibiotic use is that these powerful drugs wipe out the healthy bacteria in our gut; it's as if we took our bodies' major allies and killed them all. Suddenly our defenses are down and the bad guys have free rein.

Meanwhile, hospitals across the country worry about the rise of antibiotic resistance among bacteria. The typical hospital staff prescribes so many antibiotics that the germs that live on bedposts, monitoring equipment, sinks, doorknobs, and just about everywhere else have become resistant to most of these medical weapons. Some of the most resistant bacteria are actually resistant to *all* antibiotics, even the most powerful ones.

Certain forms of tuberculosis, for example, can no longer be cured by any known antibiotic. Bacteria such as MRSA (methicillin-resistant *Staphylococcus aureus*) and VRE (vancomycin-resistant *Enterococcus*) have developed profound resistance and represent a serious risk to patients.

Thus, taking antibiotics has the unintended consequence of instigating antibiotic resistance among the many bacteria that inhabit our gut. This process creates meaner, more invasive bacteria that are more likely to activate your immune system further.

Science has shown antibiotic use to be linked with other diseases of immune activation as well. For instance, antibiotic use in childhood increases the risk of developing asthma later in life, according to a study in *Chest* (March 2006). This report revealed that even one course of antibiotics given to children before their first birthday doubled their risk of asthma; other studies involving more than twenty-seven thousand children confirmed the finding.

Antibiotic use may also increase the risk of cancer later in life. A woman's risk of developing breast cancer was found to be more than 50 percent greater if she had a history of using antibiotics for more than fifty days in a lifetime (JAMA, February 2004).

While antibiotic use may save lives in cases of severe or life-threatening infections, too often antibiotics are prescribed in cases where our immune system can eradicate an illness on its own. Typical examples include colds, flu, sore throats, bronchitis, and even ear or sinus infections. The Centers for Disease Control and Prevention estimate that up to one-third of all U.S. antibiotic prescriptions each year are unnecessary.

DOES THE IMMUNE SYSTEM HELP OR HURT?

You may now be wondering, "Is my immune system helping me or is it killing me?"

The immune system does an outstanding job of defending us.

THE HYGIENE HYPOTHESIS

When children receive antibiotics early in life, the normal growth of desirable bacteria is destroyed. Research demonstrates that these children are more likely to develop asthma later in life, as well as develop allergies and skin conditions, and have higher rates of Crohn's disease.

Interestingly, in countries where few antibiotics are routinely prescribed (or are unavailable), scientists have found lower rates of allergies, asthma, eczema, colitis, rheumatoid arthritis, and Crohn's disease.

It's now thought that exposure to dirt, and particularly the germs found in dirt, is central to the development and function of the immune system.

There was a time when children used to come into regular contact with all the common germs, fungi, and other microbes found

But in the process, a great deal of collateral damage can occur, leading to both disease and aging.

Why does this happen? No one knows for sure, but it seems to stem from the fact that human beings are still a work in progress. There was a time—and it wasn't so long ago—when the principal cause of death was infection. Our immune system has developed over millennia to protect us from these fatal attacks.

Medical science has largely conquered infections; we have either eradicated or minimized polio, smallpox, and most of the viruses that used to kill people, with the notable exception of HIV (which specifically targets our immune system).

For those who live in developed areas of the world, the medical issues that have helped shape the evolution of the human immune system over hundreds of thousands of years are not the critical in soil. Our diets were once filled with the bacteria found in dirt; we didn't exactly eat the dirt itself, but we did eat foods that grew in it, such as carrots, potatoes, radishes, and so on. Today our food usually grows in hydroponic sterilized containers or in soil partly sterilized by pesticides and herbicides.

The single largest biomass, or the sum total weight of organic material, is found in the earth's crust—due to the huge mass of soil microorganisms within it. It seems to be important to the immune system that we commune closely with these microorganisms; if we aren't adequately exposed to them, our risk of developing allergic and autoimmune disorders increases.

The normal, close relationship between our immune system and a host of beneficial, or symbiotic, bacteria is an important one, helping to train our immune system to feel comfortable with certain outside proteins and to avoid attacking our own body. This theory, known as the hygiene hypothesis, is gaining wide recognition.

factors they once were. Today people die of heart disease, cancer, stroke, high blood pressure, kidney failure, emphysema, Alzheimer's disease—all diseases of the immune system.

Just as you are learning about the immune system by reading this book, science is learning about the immune system every day. The study of the immune system is not unlike the study of molecules. When you look closely at the latter, you see they are composed of atoms. Then you notice protons and electrons. You look still closer, and you see quarks and neutrinos; closer still, and you may find even smaller particles, and then yet smaller ones.

The immune system is similar. The closer you examine it, the more complexity you see. We certainly don't understand it fully, but we've learned more in the last decade than ever before. We now know that to live in harmony with the immune system, and to harness its power fully, we need to achieve balance. We need an immune system ready, willing, and able to fend off threats from infectious diseases, but not one that is overactive.

Read on to learn how to achieve this state of balance, this utopia of immune function and perfect health.

PART II

THE SEVEN-STEP ULTRALONGEVITY PROGRAM

SEVEN STEPS TO A STRONGER
IMMUNE SYSTEM

AS OUR PRIMARY line of defense, the immune system has evolved to respond to and protect us from any threat. The bigger the threat, the greater the response.

The immune system also works proactively, sensing our emotions and environment, and responding to even just the perception of a threat.

It's logical that our defense system should do all it can to improve our chances of survival. Lack of oxygen or water, poor nutrition, extreme stress, serious infections, and dangerous injuries can threaten our lives and evoke appropriate immune responses.

But the cost of such a response is the collateral damage that occurs in the wake of an immunologic battle. Our bodies are weakened by the threat itself as well as by our immune system's reaction to it.

The powerful and robust immune system that allowed us to survive and reproduce in a dangerous world is also the system that causes illness and aging. In an ideal world, we'd have a defense system that protected us but didn't cause any long-term harm. And that can happen—an immune system that is peaceful until needed, and is then highly responsive. But to strike this perfect balance, we must learn to control and harness the immune response. We want our immune system's power to be tempered with restraint and wisdom concerning how and when to activate.

Scientific research has identified many ways in which we can attain this. This research is the basis for the Seven-Step Ultra-Longevity Program.

Most people take a reactive approach to their health; they wait until some health problem occurs, and then, and only then, do they take action.

Taking control of your immune system means being proactive about your health; you can do this by following the steps necessary to prevent excessive immune activation rather than waiting until your immune system has run amok. Knowledge is power, and the power to control the immune system is the key to living a long, disease-free life.

In the subsequent chapters you will learn the seven easy steps needed to maintain a healthy immune system that, in turn, will thwart aging. These steps are as follows:

- **Step 1—Breathe:** Learning how to breathe properly is the first key to healthy aging. You already know breathing is important, but now you will learn more about why—and how to improve it.

- **Step 2—Eat:** It should hardly come as a surprise that your diet powerfully affects your immune system. The good news is that by following the steps in this chapter, you'll not only feel better, you'll achieve a healthy weight. Think about it—weight control and improved health at the same time!

- **Step 3—Sleep:** It's far more important to your immune system than you might have thought. Here you will learn not only why sleep is crucial, you'll discover how to sleep better.

- **Step 4—Dance:** This doesn't mean you can waltz or fox-trot your way to eternal youth, but rather that a rhythmic exercise routine can add healthy years to your life. In this chapter I'll explain why this is so and suggest new exercises you probably haven't yet considered.

- **Step 5—Love:** You don't have to be in a loving relationship with another person to experience love. Love of any kind, for anyone or anything, is the antidote for negative emotions and is good for your immune system.

- **Step 6—Soothe:** By taking steps to create a soothing environment, you and your immune system can be at peace. In this chapter you will find recommendations to enhance the world around you, and your health as well.

- **Step 7—Enhance:** Here the focus shifts from your external to your internal environment: how to bring your body and mind to peace.

Seven steps—that's all that's standing between you and a long, healthy life.

STEP 1: BREATHE

WHAT IS LIGHT as a feather, yet can't be held by even the strongest person for ten minutes?

This might be one of the oldest riddles about breath, but as far as I'm concerned, here's a much more interesting one: Why is it that breathing is one of the most essential aspects of good health, yet almost no one thinks about it? Perhaps because it is so fundamental as well as automatic.

During the course of a day, we breathe up to twenty-eight thousand times. Twenty-eight thousand times! That's approximately the same number of times that you will go to bed in your entire life—and yet how much more often do we think about sleep than about breath?

But proper breathing may well be the key to good health. The renowned osteopath and healer Dr. Robert Fulford once said, "A life is defined by breath: You take your first breath when you're born, and your last the moment you die. . . . Breath is the means by which you are connected to the universe: Without the breath, there would be no consciousness." Or as Bhante H. Gunaratana said in *Mindfulness in Plain English*, "Breathing is common to every human being, we all carry it with us everywhere we go, it is always there, constantly available, never ceasing from birth until death."

Breathing, which might seem boring and routine, is actually a complicated and remarkable process. It is such a fundamental part of life that you could even say breathing *is* life, and life is breathing. Everything living breathes: people, dogs, plants, trees, in fact, the entire planet. Breathing is the central unchanging fact of existence.

Why do we breathe? The primary reason is to exchange the gases oxygen and carbon dioxide. Normally the air we breathe in is 21 percent oxygen, and the air we breathe out is about 18 percent oxygen, meaning we extract about 3 percent of the oxygen in the air we breathe for use by our body, to help make the energy we need to function.

Meanwhile, the air we breathe in is about 0.04 percent carbon dioxide, and the air we breathe out is about 3.5 to 5 percent, depending on our level of physical exertion.

Despite the fact that we cannot live if we don't complete this exchange of oxygen and carbon dioxide, most of us don't breathe properly. We feel stressed, worried, frightened, or any number of other emotions that may cause us to hold our breath or breathe irregularly, and that's what most of us do—breathe poorly. Breathing is affected by our emotional state, and our breathing in turn affects our emotional state. It's quite common, for example, for doctors to find patients complaining of heart attack symptoms in the emergency room only to discover they are simply not breathing properly.

A classic and common example of this condition is informally known as a panic attack. Panic attacks are seldom caused by genuine panic. Most often they're caused by improper breathing.

Here's what happens: First, let's say you're feeling nervous or anxious. This causes the muscles in your chest and abdomen to become tense, which in turn restricts breathing and causes you to take faster, shallower breaths. The rapid breathing then leads to lower carbon dioxide levels in your blood, which make it harder for your body to access the oxygen carried by your blood's hemoglobin.

This process creates a vicious circle that makes you feel more tense, more anxious, and more short of breath, which then leads to even faster, shallower breaths that continue to magnify the symptoms, until you feel as if you can't breathe at all. Now you may develop chest pain or tingling in the fingers and hands. You may even pass out.

As simple as this process seems, it's so overpowering that most people find it extremely difficult to regain control of their breathing during such an attack.

The classic solution of breathing into a paper bag almost always works to halt the attack. When you rebreathe the air you exhaled into the paper bag, you are breathing in more carbon dioxide, which soon normalizes the carbon dioxide levels in your blood and overcomes the difficulty your body is having accessing oxygen. This process reverses the symptoms and effectively stops the panic attack.

By the way, improper breathing is a primary reason for the condition known as "white-coat high blood pressure." When you enter your doctor's office, you can become tense, making your breathing too shallow, which raises your heart rate and reduces heart rate variability. Your blood pressure then rises. When the doctor slaps the cuff around your arm, he or she may be alarmed at the reading. But you don't really have high blood pressure. You're just breathing poorly due to anxiety.

THREE TYPES OF BREATHING

There are three different types of breathing. The first is the most restricted kind, a breath that comes from high up in the shoulders and collarbones. You see it most often in people who are feeling panicked, or who truly are struggling for breath, as those with emphysema often do. This type of breathing is also called clavicular breathing, because it uses the collarbone (the clavicle) to help move air.

Normally our diaphragm muscle alone is responsible for inhaling. When the diaphragm (a dome-shaped, thin-layered muscle between the lungs and the abdomen) contracts, your lungs expand, pulling air in through your mouth like a bellows. When you are struggling to breathe, or your diaphragm is weak or damaged, extra muscles must be used to take over for the diaphragm. These are the muscles attached to the neck and collarbones.

Contraction of the diaphragm is triggered by the phrenic nerve, which originates in the neck—this is why, if you break a vertebra high enough up in your neck, you will not be able to breathe on your own.

Clavicular breathing, which originates from high up in the chest, neck, and shoulders, is the most abnormal form of breathing. It occurs with serious breathing impairment or during extreme stress—such as in a panic attack.

The second kind of breathing centers in the chest, and is the most common breathing pattern. People who breathe this way generally feel some stress over the course of the day and, as a result, are not breathing well—but they don't notice it. Because air is still moving in and out, they don't feel short of breath, but they are sending a message to the immune system that all is not calm.

This pattern is known as chest breathing; here, your chest will be moving, mainly upward. The muscles of your neck and collarbones are not straining, as in clavicular breathing, and the chest and lungs are expanding, but the expansion is restricted by tension and tightness in the muscles around the abdomen and ribs. This causes the chest to expand mainly upward, with less airflow and more rapid respiration.

Even though this type of breathing occurs often, especially during stress or anxiety, it almost always goes unnoticed. Breathing is an automatic process; even abnormal breathing is subconscious. Only by carefully observing your own breathing can you become mindful of your breathing technique, and only then can you correct it.

The third kind of breath comes from the abdomen, which is why it is called abdominal breathing. All of us should aspire to do it.

When breathing from your abdomen, you are more relaxed and breathing more deeply; in so doing, you are sending a message to your immune system that you are not in a state of anxiety. That important message is then transmitted throughout the body, from the brain to your heart. Your entire body now relaxes, and so does your immune system.

When you breathe from your abdomen, your belly will expand and move out with each inhalation. Your chest will rise slightly, but not nearly as much as with chest breathing. Your abdomen is doing all the moving. That's because to take in a breath, your diaphragm must contract and descend into the belly to create a vacuum effect that draws air into the lungs.

WHY WE BREATHE

People usually think that we breathe to receive oxygen, but levels of this gas are not what controls our breathing. The level of carbon dioxide in the blood primarily controls how much we breathe.

For example, when swimmers want to stay underwater for a long period of time, they hyperventilate (breathe rapidly and deeply) before jumping into the pool. This lowers the levels of carbon dioxide in the blood so it takes longer for the gas to build up and trigger the urge to breathe again, allowing a swimmer to remain underwater longer.

Only in states of severe oxygen deprivation (for example, at high altitude) does oxygen become the driver of respirations. But generally, our ability to exhale and clear carbon dioxide is the most important factor in helping to regulate our breathing.

This brings up another common misconception. Common wisdom tells us that the most important part of breathing is to get a big gulp of oxygen in a good, deep breath—but the opposite is actually the truth. The exhalation is more important. You need to focus on how you breathe out.

Our blood is quite efficient at carrying oxygen. To do this, we use hemoglobin, the compound that makes our red blood cells red. Normally, more than 95 percent of the hemoglobin in our blood is carrying oxygen. Even if this level were to drop to 85, 80, or even 70 percent, there would still be plenty of oxygen available to keep us alive.

However, if the percentage of hemoglobin carrying oxygen drops to less than 70 percent, most people will develop cyanosis, or a bluish, ghastly appearance. Still, there's quite a bit of leeway in acquiring and using oxygen, which we take in as we inhale.

Almost everyone can easily fill their lungs with air with a good, deep breath, but for people with lung diseases, getting the air out can be more challenging. For example, people who have asthma or emphysema can usually breathe in fine, but they breathe out poorly—this is when you hear them wheeze.

Sufferers of serious asthma or emphysema use a special breathing technique called pursed-lip breathing, in which they exhale through pursed or tightened lips. This helps them breathe out better, because it keeps the small airways from collapsing during a forced exhalation, when they have to push to exhale.

A full and complete deep breath out allows us to take a slow and full breath in, which slows down our respiratory cycle. Dropping our respiratory rate from twelve breaths per minute (one breath every five seconds) to six breaths a minute or less has a profound effect on our level of stress and on our immune system.

THE PHASES OF BREATHING

To be successful in gaining control of your breathing and to transmit a calm, peaceful message to your immune system, it's important to recognize and understand the four phases of breathing.

The first phase is called the inhalation phase. This is when you breathe air into your lungs.

The second phase is called the inhalation (or inspiratory) plateau, or top of the breath, which takes place after you've breathed in and before you breathe out.

Then exhalation, the third phase, begins, followed by another plateau, during which you rest. This fourth phase is called the exhalation (or expiratory) plateau, or bottom of the breath, and is the most important part of the breathing cycle. As you take in a breath, your heart rate speeds up slightly; breathe out and your heart rate slows slightly. At the bottom of the breath, in the expiratory plateau, your heart rate is at its slowest, and you can feel the overall sense of well-being associated with this level of relaxation.

Let's examine these phases. When you start breathing, it feels good to take in a breath. But as you continue to breathe, your chest will feel full, until you can't breathe anymore. When you get to the full expansion of the chest, you feel a little discomfort or uneasiness; your brain tells you to stop breathing in.

You're now at the inspiratory plateau, where you feel comfortable for only a moment before you're hit with the urge to breathe out. So you do, and it feels good. When done, you've come to the exhalation plateau, when the chest muscles and diaphragm are relaxed and most of the air is out of your lungs.

There is an essential feeling of repose that occurs in the initial part of the exhalation plateau. But if you stay there too long, you feel tension again. Now you want to take another breath in.

This back-and-forth state of tension and relaxation happens twelve to twenty times a minute, depending on how fast you breathe; it's a fascinating microcosm of the struggle in life between stress and peace.

Once you've recognized and begun to understand the four phases of breathing, spend a few minutes sensing and cherishing each of the phases and the alternating pleasure and tension that happens with each breath. Also, recognize the very special peace you feel in the exhalation plateau at the bottom of each breath.

BREATHING AND YOUR HEALTH

When people aren't breathing properly, a few things occur. Let's say you're feeling threatened. Your muscles become tense. This tension starts to impede your breathing, tightening the muscles of your chest and belly. You can't get a full, deep breath when you feel this anxious. Instead, your breathing becomes restricted, and whenever that happens, the immune system senses a threat.

Our immune system wants as much early warning about threats as possible so it can gear up to protect us. That's its job. So when that early warning comes in the form of shallow or restricted breathing, the immune system gets to work, signals the forces, and prepares for battle.

There is a new body of research that shows that all of the breathing disorders, from asthma to tuberculosis, from emphysema to interstitial lung diseases, have been linked with an overactive immune system.

More than a dozen recent studies have confirmed the link between impaired breathing and immune activation. The conclusion of these studies, as reported in *Thorax* in March 2004, was that reduced lung function was associated with systemic immune activation as measured by white blood counts and levels of CRP and TNF-alpha.

It's no surprise, then, that a twenty-nine-year study of longevity (the Buffalo Health Study) showed that pulmonary function and breathing capacity were excellent predictors of long-term survival for both men and women (*Chest*, March 2000).

And in another study of twenty-one volunteers who were to

practice a mindful breathing technique, immune function, as measured by natural killer cell activity, was shown to improve after subjects attended a breathing class and learned mindful breathing (*Journal of Alternative and Complementary Medicine*, April 2005).

The immune system is not the only system to benefit from proper breathing. The brain benefits as well. Research from Japan (published in *Neuroscience Research* in November 2004) shows that during relaxed abdominal breathing, brain waves also show a pattern of relaxation—that is, they show a shift to a slower, more rhythmic pattern. Deliberate and mindful breathing creates a slow and organized brain-wave pattern observable on an electroencephalograph (EEG). This synchronization between the breath and the brain or other systems has been called entrainment, and rhythmic harmony is also transmitted to the heart.

One of the ways we measure the level of entrainment of breathing and heartbeat is by measuring the pulse—but not in the usual way. Normally, when you check a pulse, you're getting an average heart rate for thirty or sixty seconds. A more precise way to measure pulse rate is to carefully measure the interval from one beat to the next. If you take a good look at the heart this way, precisely measuring the intervals between beats for a full minute, you'll see that a healthy heartbeat varies widely. That beat-to-beat variation in heart rate is called heart rate variability (HRV).

You would think you'd want your heartbeat to be very regular. Actually, that's dangerous. The more regular someone's heartbeat is, the sicker he or she is.

In fact, the sickest person might be someone who had a bad heart, underwent a heart transplant, and now has a new heart in his or her body. This person's heart rate tends to be 100 percent regular, with no variability at all—which is not good. A transplanted heart is cut off from most of its normal connections; nerves that normally control the heart rate have been severed, so a transplanted heart receives very few signals about how fast it should be beating. In fact, an artificial pacemaker is often installed just to give the transplanted heart more variability.

Heart rate variability has been studied extensively. Poor HRV has been linked with increased mortality after heart attack (*Journal of Cardiovascular Electrophysiology*, January 2005), and has also been shown to be linked with depression, anger, and anxiety. And in a study of 643 healthy men and women in Denmark, reported in the *European Heart Journal* in December 2003, reduced heart rate variability was linked with immune activation, as measured by CRP and white blood count levels.

In other words, the poorer the HRV, the more hyperactivated the immune system. However, proper breathing can improve heart rate variability and reduce immune activation.

The youngest and healthiest people—kids—have an extremely variable heart rate; it's all over the map. That's very healthy. The connections between a child's heart and his or her brain and breathing are quite strong, and so every breath causes a predictable variation in the heart rate.

This variability relates to the breath cycle. As you breathe in, your heart rate speeds up, and as you breathe out, your heart rate slows down.

Heart rate variability can be measured fairly easily with a specialized heart rate monitor that precisely measures the beat-to-beat heart rate and plots it over time.

Consumer products are now available to help train people to improve their heart rate variability using breathing and biofeedback. For more information, check out www.freezeframer.com.

The bottom line: when we consciously and mindfully focus on our breathing, a rhythmic pattern of healthy heart rate variability and healthy immune function result. And that means a longer and healthier life.

TAKE ACTION: BREATHE

There's plenty of additional evidence linking labored or impaired breathing with the activation of the immune system and lung diseases such as emphysema, asthma, and bronchitis. Equally important, when these conditions are treated, an improvement in immune system functioning nearly always occurs.

Learning to breathe properly is one way everyone can support their immune system. The good news is that there are many things you can do to improve breathing, and therefore your immune system.

BECOME AWARE

Perhaps the most important way to take care of your breath is simply to become more aware of it. Once you do, you may be amazed to discover how disordered your breathing actually is.

Right now, even as you are reading this, pay attention to your body. Become aware of the tension in the muscles of your chest, neck, shoulders, and abdomen. Pay particular attention to the belly, which should be expanding freely with each breath in.

What you're likely to discover is that you often hold your breath, you breathe irregularly, and/or your breath stutters. Many patterns of breathing are pathological, including a condition known as Cheyne-Stokes respiration, a common breathing pattern characterized by alternating periods of apnea and hyperpnea; in other words, the breather alternates between very slow or absent breathing and deep, rapid breathing every minute or so.

Unlike heart monitors, breath monitors are not yet widely available (although we are currently working on a small device that will help people monitor their breathing habits). Until they are, here are the best ways to monitor your breath.

1. **Pay attention to the four stages of breathing:** Inhalation, plateau, exhalation, plateau. The objective is to prolong exhalation and the exhalation plateau. Appreciate and enjoy the peaceful relaxation of the expiratory plateau.

   If you time your breathing, you should find that the ratio of inhalation to exhalation is approximately one to two: the exhalation should take twice as long as the inhalation, with the exhalation plateau longer than the inhalation plateau. Someone who breathes very well can make that exhalation plateau last quite a long time. This can be uncomfortable for some people, but if you are feeling good, it can be very peaceful. An experienced practitioner can stay in the exhalation plateau for thirty seconds or more.

   During breathing exercises, your goal should be slow, paced breathing. In a state of relaxation, the respiratory rate can drop as low as two to three breaths per minute. This translates to allowing seven to ten seconds for a breath in (including the inspiratory plateau), and fourteen to twenty seconds for the breath out (including the expiratory plateau).

2. **Feel the breath:** One simple way to check on your breathing is to fold your arms across your belly while you're sitting. With each breath in, your arms should rise and move upward. That means your abdomen is expanding and you are performing abdominal breathing. If your arms don't move up, or if they move inward, you need to focus on relaxing and expanding your belly with each breath.

   Another way to help increase awareness of your breathing is to place your right hand on your upper abdomen and your left hand on your upper chest. You should feel your right hand moving out and away from your spine with each inhalation, while your left hand remains fairly stationary or moves outward just slightly.

If your right hand is stationary or moving inward with each breath and your left hand is moving up and outward, then you are experiencing chest or clavicular breathing. Concentrate on relaxing your belly and using each breath to expand your belly outward. Continue with this as slowly as is comfortable.

3. **Focus on breathing:** If you find you are having difficulty mastering this, try adding some thoughts that will help you focus.

With each breath in, think the word *energy*.

With each breath out, think the word *relax*.

Say each word to yourself with each breath; use them as a mantra to help focus your breathing. Pause after each word at the top and bottom of each breath long enough to bask in the plateau phases.

IMPROVE YOUR BREATHING MECHANICS

The best way to tell your immune system that things are okay is to breathe properly, so here are some suggestions on how to do it.

1. **Add physical exercise:** Vigorous physical exercise will force you to breathe deeply and move air through your body. Almost any exercise will do: walk, run, jog, bowl, dance, roller blade, or ice skate. Even walking up stairs at home or up hills around your neighborhood can help. Your goal is simply to add a daily routine of any exercise that strengthens your breathing.

2. **Breathe against resistance:** You might think that the best way to train your breathing is through activities such as blowing up a balloon—and yes, this is good practice. However, the muscles we use to breathe in (our diaphragm) tend to be weaker than the muscles we use to blow up a balloon (our chest wall and abdominal muscles).

It's similar to the way the rest of the muscles in your body work—your quads are stronger than your hamstrings, your biceps are stronger than your triceps. In other words, flexion tends to be stronger than extension. When your arms are flexed, they're stronger than when they're extended. The same is true of breathing. There are many muscles you can use to exhale—all the muscles around the chest, and even the belly. But only one muscle can make you inhale air—the diaphragm.

Since most people can blow up a balloon well, slightly more difficult exercises will involve sucking rather than blowing.

For example, in hospitals, doctors reconditioning patients to breathe better will place them on a routine of sucking exercises, such as using a small device requiring the patient to suck air from a resistant straw; a little ball inside the transparent device indicates how forcefully he or she is using the diaphragm.

An easy way to do this at home: Make a fist, and then place your fist in front of your mouth and inhale through the fist; the smaller the hole you create in your fist, the harder it is to suck the air. While you're breathing in against the resistance created by your fist, concentrate on your abdomen and diaphragm, making sure your belly is expanding with each breathe inward.

Do this for four or five breaths twice a day, but don't do these exercise breaths all in a row; alternate them with normal breaths. Otherwise, you're really just practicing holding your breath rather than strengthening your diaphragm.

Another at-home idea is to use an incentive spirometer. Doctors often prescribe this inexpensive device to help patients recover more quickly from surgery, or to help improve breathing after pneumonia or bronchitis. You can buy it at your local drugstore for about ten dollars. Incentive spirometers provide resistance to inspiration that helps condition the diaphragm.

3. **Sigh:** Yes—sigh. If your breathing feels tense, jittery, or stiff, incorporate a few sighs into your day. Sighing creates a bit more

resistance to airflow on exhalation, and this can help relax the chest muscles.

To help relax muscles in the chest and abdomen and correct jittery breathing, first take a full, deep breath in through your nose so that your lungs are completely filled. Then exhale, and while the air is exiting, say "Aaaahhhhh" softly in a sighing sound.

Repeat this three times in succession and your chest and abdominal muscles should relax.

4. **Swim:** The kind of rhythmic breathing required when swimming the crawl, for example, can help build lung capacity while also pacing your breathing. Swimmers develop tremendous lung capacity through the regular exercise of breathing as they move through the water.

5. **Try RESPeRATE:** RESPeRATE is a portable device that provides sounds that cue you to breathe at a set pace. It can help improve the cadence of breathing and can even help lower blood pressure. RESPeRATE is available online at www.resperate.com.

6. **Sing, or play a wind instrument:** Singing, or playing the flute, saxophone, or other wind instruments, requires breath control. If you can't sing or play an instrument, then try whistling. These are all enjoyable ways to improve your breathing technique, and you will also gain from the therapeutic effect music has on the immune system (see the Soothe step).

7. **Go online:** Many excellent Web sites provide instruction or products relating to breathing and health, including www.breathing .com, www.buteyko.com, www.nishinojuku.com/english/e_top .html, www.resperate.com, and www.freezeframer.com.

STEP 2: EAT

- *The toughest part of a diet isn't watching what you eat. It's watching what other people eat.*
- *You know you have to go on a diet when you're diagnosed with the flesh-eating virus and the doctor gives you thirty more years to live.*
- *Did you hear about the guy who went on a diet, swore off drinking and heavy eating, and in fourteen days he lost two weeks?*
- *How about the beggar who tells a woman entering a coffee shop that he hasn't eaten in a week? The woman says, "I wish I had your willpower."*

THERE ARE PROBABLY as many diet jokes out there as there are kinds of diets. Yet dieting isn't very funny—nor is finding the best way to make smart food choices.

Most people realize that eating food provides them with energy, vitamins, and minerals. But what few know is that food is also an extremely important signal to the immune system—and therefore the aging process.

The immune system responds to eating in many different ways—and not just to the specific food you happen to be consuming, but also to the pattern of your eating, the way you eat, where you eat, and even with whom you eat.

Each of these cues has its own impact on the immune system. For example, drinking a glass of wine over dinner with friends has a very different effect than downing a bottle alone while you're working at your computer. Likewise, eating a nutritious, calm breakfast with your partner sends your immune system a different message from the one it receives when you're having an equally nutritious but anxiety-charged breakfast with your boss.

Although eating is a broad topic, when it comes to the immune system, there are six main areas to consider: hunger, eating patterns, emotional eating, the quantity of food you eat, your eating environment, and digestion.

HUNGER

Few people nowadays rely on hunger as their impetus to eat. Instead, our cue is a social event, a dinner reservation, or feelings such as boredom, depression, anxiety, or stress. Many of my patients never experience hunger at all. They'll even admit, "I can't remember the last time I was hungry."

But you should feel a little bit hungry every three hours or so— not a sense of starvation, but a reminder that your body is ready for refueling. A gentle signal to eat something every few hours means the balance of hunger hormones in your body is just about right. For the most part, people who don't experience hunger eat too much.

A number of hormones produce the sensation of appetite; scientific research is just beginning to learn about them. In the future, you will likely hear much more about leptin, ghrelin, adiponectin, obestatin, and other hormones yet to be discovered.

The research suggests that hormones exert a powerful impact on the immune system, and that the sensation of hunger may actually be one way the body lets us feel how well our immune system is functioning.

Leptin, for example, is critical for maintaining weight. It shuts off appetite and tells your brain when you have eaten enough. Leptin also increases your metabolism and makes you burn more calories. So it would seem that having lots of leptin around would be good—anything that lowers appetite and boosts metabolism could also help promote weight loss.

In reality, however, thin people have lower leptin levels, while overweight people have higher ones. This makes sense when you understand that leptin is produced by fat cells, and that its purpose is to regulate appetite and weight. So if you gain weight (fat), more leptin is produced, appetite goes down, and metabolism goes up. This process has the effect of encouraging the body to shed pounds and return to your original weight.

Conversely, if you lose weight, your leptin levels drop, but your appetite then increases and metabolism slows. This process tends to make you gain back the lost weight, again returning to where you started. I'm sure many of you are familiar with this pattern; it's a built-in, protective function designed to maintain your weight at a set point.

Research indicates that leptin has a powerful effect on the immune system—namely, activating it. Thus people who are thin, with lower leptin levels, have less immune activation, while overweight people, with higher levels of leptin, show more immune activation—and will probably suffer from more immune system problems such as arthritis, diabetes, heart disease, high blood pressure, and cancer.

We now understand that immune activation caused by leptin and the other hunger hormones is one of the main reasons obesity has been linked with so many different diseases.

EATING PATTERNS

Eating patterns are another important health consideration. Patterns of eating vary according to our familial, cultural, ethnic, and professional background. People who work night shifts, for example, eat differently from people who work nine to five. Those who come from large families have different eating patterns than those from smaller families, and so on.

Current medical research now suggests that in many cases of obesity where most, if not all, of the members of the patient's family are overweight, the culprit is rarely an inherited obesity gene. Rather, the trait passed on seems related to eating pattern behavior; if your parents often ate large meals or frequent junk-food snacks, most likely you do too.

Many of the most common eating patterns reflect emotional issues. People who become anxious when alone in the evening are apt to adopt an eating pattern intended to soothe their anxiety. Using comfort foods such as brownies, cookies, or cheeseburgers to pacify the soul can lead to a habit of munching that begins before a stressful day and ends with a midnight snack. And this, of course, leads directly to immune stimulation.

Whichever of the many different eating patterns you follow, what matters most is that you recognize the pattern and understand its impact on your health.

Most people can intuitively identify these patterns because they've been following them all their lives. For example, if you're not a morning person, you tend to skip breakfast, eat a late lunch, and sit down to dinner when other folks are going to bed. This pattern means that you're getting about 80 percent of your daily calories after 4 p.m.

As you now know, eating the bulk of your daily calories in one meal overstimulates the immune system and causes a mini aging spurt. Changing your pattern of eating to spread calorie consumption over the course of the day is one way to curtail this process.

Of course, it's not always easy to alter these patterns. One of the questions I'm most frequently asked is, "Doc, I'm not hungry when I get up in the morning. Should I eat anyway?"

The real issue isn't what you should or shouldn't do when you get up. It's that a person who isn't hungry in the morning probably ate her breakfast for dinner the night before—in other words, she continued to eat after 9 or 10 p.m., enjoying a sizable snack, probably loaded with quick carbohydrates and too many calories. Of course she has no appetite when she wakes up.

The way to shake someone out of this habit is to ask her to eat breakfast when she rises in the morning. What she'll usually find is that when she does, she's hungry again at midday and will eat lunch. By the time dinner rolls around, she won't have her normal appetite because she's been eating correctly throughout the day; that late night craving should also diminish.

Like our body temperature and our metabolism rate, our appetite has its own thermostat that tells us when to eat. The appetite thermostat is set to shut off when we have eaten enough daily calories to maintain our current weight. So if the bulk of those calories have been eaten by three o'clock in the afternoon, you'll have a smaller appetite at dinner and later.

Also, if you supplement your diet with a few small, low-calorie snacks during the day, you'll decrease your appetite in the evening and will end up eating less—and wake up the next morning feeling hungry. This habit helps perpetuate a healthy eating pattern.

EMOTIONAL EATING

As we touched on earlier, emotional eating is another common diet-related concern. For most people, eating produces a state of calm, satisfaction, or even mild euphoria, for reasons having to do with chemistry and survival. Despite our well-stocked refrigerators, our genes are still geared toward locating food and eating it, among the most primal of all survival instincts. And eating causes a release of serotonin, one of our calm-inducing neurotransmitters. So naturally, if you're not feeling well, you'll instinctively reach for food. Food numbs tension, anxiety, fright, and despair.

FOOD, AGE, AND ALLERGIES

The point in your life at which you first ingest specific foods exerts an important effect on your immune system. For example, first eating grains when you're five months old has a different effect on your immune system than first eating them when you're five years old.

Remember, your immune system is constantly touching, identifying, and processing information about the myriad foreign proteins with which you come into contact every day. New proteins are constantly being checked against the cumulative database of threats stored in the memory of more than a billion B cells floating through your bloodstream. That database is being created as soon as you are born, with new entries added every minute of the day. We call this process the learning feature of your adaptive immune system.

Early in life is also when, if an item is "misfiled" in the database, it can make a lasting impact. One fairly common filing error occurs during the vulnerable period between about three and six months of age, when your immune system just begins learning.

This is actually contradictory, because while you may feel that you are calming your emotions, in reality you're hyping your immune system. The poor thing now has to get busy sorting through all that funky food to check whether any invaders have crawled in with it. This activation is why emotional eating is one of the most common hazards of our relationship to food.

One of the easy exercises we recommend to overcome emotional eating is the hunger check. Simply put, we want you to eat because you're hungry, not because you're anxious, mad, or sad.

The hunger check is a powerful way to discover the emotional basis of eating. Each time a fork or spoon is poised to enter your mouth, pause for just a second and ask yourself, "Am I hungry right now?"

If the answer is yes, go right ahead and enjoy!

Before three months of age, your immunity depends largely on the information passed on to it from your mother through the placenta and then in breast milk. Maternal antibodies (made by your mother's immune system) are transferred through the blood and breast milk to protect you against threats you might encounter in the first few weeks of life.

By the time you're about three months old, however, your immune system has matured enough to begin to create antibodies and store memories on its own. During this highly sensitive period, exposure to the wrong foreign protein can produce unwanted effects. For example, when babies are fed their first grains at between three and six months, the odds of their developing autoimmune diseases such as type 1 diabetes and celiac disease (gluten allergy) rise considerably.

Thus it's very important to be aware of this vulnerability when we feed our children—grains are best introduced into a baby's diet a bit later, at between six and nine months of age.

If the answer is no, the next question should be, "Then why am I about to eat this?"

The answer to this second question is likely to be that you are experiencing an emotional state such as tension, anxiety, anger, melancholy, or even boredom.

QUANTITY OF FOOD

When it comes to the immune system, the quantity of food you eat is as important as the quality. The reason? The greater the quantity of food you ingest in a single meal, the more strain you place on your immune system.

Researchers measuring after-meal CRP levels in test subjects have found that the higher the meal's caloric content, the higher the CRP level afterward. This means that people who eat smaller, more frequent meals have a milder immune system reaction than those who eat all of their daily calories in a few big meals.

Why is that? Scientists aren't yet sure, but one of the most credible theories derives from the fact that, as mentioned, a large portion of our immune system resides in the gut, patrolling the gastrointestinal tract, which is one of the major entry points for germs, microbes, and other threats. Each time we swallow anything, the immune system activates its sentries to scan the borders and make sure nothing is trying to penetrate them.

Through the process of digestion, the food we eat is broken down into smaller and smaller molecules to be absorbed by our small intestines. Ideally, large complex proteins should be digested completely, down to their component building blocks, known as amino acids. Proteins have an inherent ability to stimulate our immune system and cause a reaction, whereas amino acids do not; the latter aren't large or complex enough to trigger one.

But the process that allows for the absorption of food also allows for invaders to cross the gut membrane, the barrier between the gut and our body.

There's been a great deal of research into these invaders, known as antigens, which traverse the lining of the gut and, in so doing, activate the immune system. In fact, approximately 2 percent of all the food antigens we ingest successfully cross the gut membrane.

Once these antigens have entered our body, they have a much greater chance of causing an immune response. This process is one of the ways that people develop food allergies.

If 2 percent of food antigens we eat are able to enter our system and cause an immune reaction, then the larger the meal, the greater the likelihood of immune activation. So simply by eating a large quantity of food, we supply a strong stimulant to the immune system.

This research helps to explain why so much of the data on aging shows that the restriction of calorie intake has a profound effect on the aging process—to the point that if a laboratory mouse's calorie intake is reduced by about a third, the mouse will live 30 or 40 percent longer than it would in nature. In human terms, if you take our current life span of about seventy-five to eighty years and increase that by 30 to 40 percent, you'd get an average life span of about one hundred years!

More and more, it seems that one of the ways to live a long, healthy life is by reducing the quantity of food we eat, or more specifically, calorie restriction. So far, experiments on many animal species confirm the effect of calorie restriction on longevity. Mice, rats, hamsters, fruit flies, monkeys, baboons, and chimps all live longer if they're fed fewer calories than normal.

However, a problem arises when people are asked to eat fewer calories: the psychology of deprivation. It takes machinelike discipline for people to maintain low-calorie food intake. When you feel deprivation, all kinds of negative emotions follow. You feel terrible about it, you can't think about anything else. If you cheat, you feel guilty. Or if you succeed for a length of time, you may reward yourself so generously that you eat more than you ever did before.

On the UltraLongevity program, we encourage the opposite approach. We tell people to eat *more* frequently—as long as they are eating foods that are low in calories.

By constantly eating more low-calorie foods, and getting that feeling of being full without having consumed a great many calories, we can avoid activation of the immune system.

Most people are already aware of this psychological technique. For example, you know that when you're going to a late dinner, by the time you get there and order your meal, you'll be so hungry you'll devour two appetizers, a basket of bread, and dinner, as well as two drinks, dessert, and maybe the tablecloth too. So instead you eat a salad beforehand to avoid being ravenous later.

The ideal pattern of eating is as follows: Graze whenever you feel hungry. Eat frequently, but take in fewer calories. When you eat this way, you should feel full—and your immune system will not be overworked.

Every three hours, you should notice that you're starting to get a little hungry. When that happens, you can munch on a low-calorie snack (and I mean a snack, such as a handful of raisins or peanuts, not a meal). Three hours later, you're probably hungry again. And again you have a low-calorie snack.

By eating small amounts of food more frequently, you prevent the surges of immune activation that follow large meals. In fact, you could say that every large meal creates an aging spurt that cumulatively accelerates the clock by activating your immune system. But a sustainable eating strategy that effectively reduces the total intake of calories and the immune activation that follows a large meal reduces the speed of aging.

EATING ENVIRONMENT

The setting in which you eat also matters.

Too many people eat while driving their cars, or standing up at counters, or working at their desks. This isn't just potentially messy, it's unhealthy. Eating in such unpleasant ways increases your level of stress, and that's hardly kind to your immune system.

As you've learned, each time you eat, your immune system mobilizes its forces to make sure you haven't ingested some dangerous enemy. If you heap a high level of stress on top of the activity of eating, the immune system gears up even more.

You should always eat while sitting down, in a calm environment dedicated to just that: eating. And don't eat while juggling two or three other things. Multitasking is a wonderful skill, but not at the dinner table.

Of course, it's not always possible to eat in the right setting— modern life is too hectic. But whenever you can, make the effort to eat in a social environment. Just as social networks reduce immune activation, so can social networking over meals.

Unfortunately, many American families have lost the ritual of the family dinner. In Europe, the value placed on meals as a focus of social gatherings still exists. Such social connections improve digestion and reduce the stress of eating on the immune system. This may in part explain the so-called French paradox—somehow the French manage to eat meals high in saturated fat but don't develop heart disease at nearly the same rate as Americans do.

DIGESTION

Strangely, few people think about digestion while they're eating, even though if it weren't for digestion, there would be no point to eating at all. Digestion is the only way we can turn food into the energy and basic raw materials we need for growth, functioning, and repair of the body.

During the process of digestion, complex foods are systematically broken down into their component building blocks, which our bodies then use for various purposes. Fuels such as fats and sugars are either burned immediately or stored for our future energy needs, DNA is broken down into its component nucleotides, and proteins are digested into their respective building blocks, the amino acids.

Our body uses twenty different amino acids, from which we can construct thousands upon thousands of different proteins. Many of them are unique to human beings, and a few may even be unique to individuals. These proteins vary in size, from a strand of just a few amino acids (in the case of a protein called a polypeptide) to many thousands of amino acids strung together like beads on a necklace.

The specific sequence of amino acids is what makes each protein unique and also what gives it a three-dimensional structure, rendering it capable of performing special functions in the body.

Our immune system does not react to amino acids but to chains

ELIMINATION DIETS

When a patient's immune system is up in arms, we must consider whether certain foods may be contributing to his or her immune activation. Some clues might include such postmeal symptoms as bloating, stomach pain, itchy skin, flushing, excessive gas, cramps, soreness, or fatigue. Or unexplained activation of the immune system may take place, causing arthritis, colitis, or psoriasis, for instance. Sometimes blood testing can show high levels of antibodies in response to specific foods. In such situations, we recommend patients try an elimination diet.

During an elimination diet, all possible food triggers are removed from the diet for at least ten weeks and the effect is observed. It's not always easy to know which foods need to be eliminated; blood testing can be somewhat helpful, but it's by no means foolproof or exact.

Instead, we ask people to eliminate the foods most likely to be causing a reaction, such as dairy, wheat- and gluten-containing foods, nuts, shellfish, eggs, and soy.

Take Daria, for example. Forty-four years old, Daria had been feeling sick for a dozen years. Her doctors had diagnosed her with fibromyalgia, lupus, and autoimmune thyroid disease.

Two years before we met, Daria had had to stop working as an interior designer because of extreme fatigue, generalized pain, and unpleasant, electric shock–like sensations coursing through her body. Daria's mother had lived for years with multiple sclerosis, and Daria feared hearing the same diagnosis that had left her mother disabled and wheelchair bound.

When we performed blood tests, we found Daria's immune

system seriously overactivated—so much so that her doctors had placed her on high doses of a steroid (prednisone) and gobs of pain-killers, none of which was really helping.

When I first met Daria, her CRP level was 6.3 (it should be less than 0.7) and her white blood count was 11.7 (it should be around 5). Her sed rate was elevated at 29 (normal is about 10) and her cholesterol level was 467!

Needless to say, neither Daria nor I was happy with these results. So our first step was to put Daria on an elimination diet. She quickly removed dairy, gluten, soy, shellfish, eggs, and nuts from her meals. Initially, Daria found this a tough task, because these were some of her favorite foods; curling up on the sofa with a pasta dinner was her idea of pure comfort. But her health was so poor she was motivated to try anything. She also hated her medications and their side effects.

In addition, Daria concentrated on thorough chewing, quantity control, eating pattern, and all the other important techniques for proper eating.

The goal of this process was to reduce the quantity of food antigens that were crossing the lining of her digestive tract and potentially causing her immune system to react. She wasn't technically allergic to any of the forbidden foods; they were simply causing immune activation.

By following this program, within eight weeks Daria was able to get off of prednisone and she lost sixteen pounds. Thrilled, she continued the program. Six months later she had lost thirty-one pounds. A year later, her CRP was down to 0.8, her white blood count and thyroid hormone levels were normal, and her cholesterol was down to 191.

of amino acids strung together into proteins. Proteins from other organisms, whether from plants or animals, are recognized by our immune system as potential invaders. For example, the proteins on the surface of a staph bacterium, a herpesvirus, an amoeba, or any other parasite are viewed as foreign and possibly dangerous.

One objective of our digestive tract is to break down the immune-stimulating, foreign proteins we eat into safe, nonreactive amino acid building blocks so that we can use these to build our own proteins.

If our digestive tract doesn't work properly and foreign proteins enter our bloodstream, our immune system will be exposed to, and react to, these proteins every time we eat.

To prevent such a major immune reaction every time we eat, we need to digest our food properly. Digestion is a multipart process that begins with salivation and chewing. In fact, the act of merely thinking about food has an effect on your immune system; most of us have felt that enormous sense of anticipation that arises from just knowing a great meal is in the offing.

Once you place the food in your mouth, your saliva, which contains the enzyme amylase, helps break down starch, while chewing increases the surface area of the food, which in turn helps the enzymes in our saliva, stomach, pancreas, and liver to do their jobs more effectively.

When the food arrives inside our stomach, the digestive process continues. The stomach churns to help further break down the food, while the cells lining it produce hydrochloric acid to break food down even more. Hydrochloric acid also activates strong enzymes known as proteases, such as pepsin and trypsin, which cleave amino acids from protein chains like snipping the links of a sausage.

Our pancreas and liver are involved in digestion too. The pancreas makes enzymes including lipase and amylase, and the liver produces bile, which emulsifies fats.

This complex but well-designed system kicks in every time we eat, whether it's a small snack or a Thanksgiving dinner. Too often, though, people bolt down their food rather than chew it well. When you do that, you end up with a big blob of protein stuck in your stomach. Your system must now rely on stomach acid and enzymes alone to break it down into all its component parts.

Nearly every gastroenterologist in the country has had to put a scope down the stomach of someone who ate too quickly and swallowed such a big piece of meat it got stuck in the esophagus. It won't go down, it won't come back up—the only recourse is for the doctor and his or her gastroscope to go on a fishing expedition.

So remember, from the standpoint of your immune system, digestion is critical to prevent an immune reaction every time you eat—and unless you thoroughly chew your food, proper digestion doesn't take place.

WHAT TO EAT

What you eat is as important as how you eat it. That's why you must make informed choices. For instance, you should eat fish twice a week due to its DHA content. DHA, or docosahexaenoic acid, is one of the beneficial omega-3 fats. Research shows that the higher your DHA level, the lower your CRP level. Eating fish a couple times a week (and perhaps supplementing it with DHA pills) is an excellent strategy to help reduce immune activation. (We'll talk more about DHA supplements in the Enhance chapter.)

As most people now know, your best choice is fish that haven't been exposed to an overabundance of contaminants, such as mercury. These fish tend to be wild rather than farm-raised fish. They also tend to come from the smaller species, as the larger ones build up a greater concentration of contaminants in their bodies. Among the smaller wild fish: wild salmon, arctic char, sole, mackerel, herring, sardines, and nonfarmed trout.

In contrast, swordfish are large and accumulate many contaminants. Even the big tuna that are made into sushi or tuna steaks may contain too many pollutants to be suitable for regular consumption—further research is still needed to determine what levels, if any, are safe.

Nuts are also important to support your immune system (as long as you're not allergic). They're a rich source of vitamin E and contain beneficial fat and minerals such as selenium, a powerful immune system suppressant. Just two Brazil nuts a day fulfills your daily selenium requirement.

Also enjoy the healthy oils. Olive oil, especially the extra-virgin, first-cold-pressed oil, should be your first choice, rather than corn, safflower, or sunflower oils. However, canola oil can be a reasonable substitute, especially if it's the cold-pressed canola oil available in your natural food store rather than that sold at grocery stores and shopping centers, which has often been heated or chemically extracted with hexane.

Then, of course, there's broccoli and its family, the cruciferous vegetables. These include cauliflower, cabbage, kale, bok choy, brussels sprouts, broccolini, and kohlrabi. All of these foods possess an important ingredient for the immune system called sulforaphane.

Fiber, too, is crucial; much research has linked high-fiber diets with low immune activation. The higher your intake of dietary fiber, the lower your CRP. The reason for this pattern seems to be that fiber encourages the growth of symbiotic bacteria—organisms with which we live in harmony—such as acidophilus and bifidobacteria and some forms of E. coli. Fiber is their food; they live on it. And as mentioned, these friendly inhabitants support our own immune system.

How much fiber should you eat? Most people should get about twenty grams of dietary fiber for every 1,000 calories consumed in a day. So if you're eating 1,500 daily calories, you should shoot for thirty grams of dietary fiber.

Some of the great fiber-rich foods include whole grains, such as whole wheat, brown rice, whole oats, millet, and quinoa. Then there are the already mentioned nuts and seeds, and the legume family, including lentils, split peas, kidney beans, and snap peas. Many other vegetables and fruits are good sources of dietary fiber. (In the Enhance step, we'll talk about how to supplement your diet to achieve your fiber goals.)

IMMUNE-FRIENDLY FOODS

Following is a list of some of the foods and spices that best reduce immune activation. These foods should be eaten often; spices should be added liberally. Think of them as the closest thing to a fountain of youth in your grocery store.

CATEGORY	EXAMPLES	NUTRIENTS
Garlic family	Garlic, onions, scallions, shallots, chives, leeks	Trisulfides, allicin, S-allylcysteine
Berries	Raspberries, blackberries, black raspberries, loganberries, blueberries, bilberries, cranberries, huckleberries	Gallic acid, sanguiin H-6, proanthocyanidins, flavonols, anthocyanins
Fruits, melons	Apples, pears, quince, cherries, apricots, plums, peaches, etc.; watermelon, cantaloupe, papaya	Quercetin, proanthocyanidins, lycopene
Nightshades	Tomatoes, especially tomato sauce, tomatillos, eggplant, cayenne, chili peppers	Lycopene, nasunin (anthocyanin), capsaicin
Grapes	Grapes, wine	Resveratrol, grapeseed extract
Small fish	Salmon, arctic char, sole, trout, herring, mackerel, sardines	DHA (docosahexaenoic acid), EPA (eicosapentaenoic acid)

CATEGORY	EXAMPLES	NUTRIENTS
Nuts, seeds	Walnuts, almonds, pecans, cashews, hazelnuts, Brazil nuts, etc.	Selenium, monounsaturated fats
Citrus	Oranges, lemons, limes, grapefruits, tangerines, etc.	Bioflavonoids, d-limonene
Brewed beverages	Coffee, teas	Polyphenols, catechins, xanthines, zeaxanthins, theanine
Cruciferous vegetables and leafy greens	Broccoli, cabbage, brussels sprouts, cauliflower, kale, collard greens, Swiss chard, spinach, mustard greens, etc.	Lutein, folate, sulforaphane
Root crops and pumpkins	Carrots, squash, yams/sweet potatoes, pumpkins	Carotene
Herbs and spices	Basil, turmeric, rosemary	Curcumin, polyphenols
Olives	Olives and olive oil	Monounsaturated fat, polyphenols

TAKE ACTION: EAT

FOLLOW THE CHECK LIST

By adopting healthier eating patterns, you can help reduce immune activation and live in harmony with your diet. The best way to do so is to follow what I call a five-point CHECK List:

1. **Chew check:** Are you chewing enough so that the food is almost liquefied before you swallow? If you need to, you can even count the number of times you chew (such as twenty-five), but

that shouldn't be necessary. Just remind yourself to slow down and completely chew each bite.

2. **Hunger check:** Before you put food into your mouth, pause and ask yourself if you are truly hungry. If the answer is yes, eat. If the answer is no, put down your fork, breathe, take a sip of water, and consider doing something else.

3. **Emotion check:** Be aware that you're eating. That alone should make you happy; you should be calm and breathing easily, rather than pressured or stressed. Sense the muscles of your brow and face—are they relaxed? Are you smiling, or at least not scowling? If not, remind yourself how wonderful it is to be able to sit peacefully and eat, to take a break and just savor your meal.

4. **Company check:** Did you invite someone to eat with you, or has someone invited you? Try to make at least one meal a day a social gathering. Enjoy the company of a friend or loved one while you eat and your immune system will thank you.

5. **Kcal (kilocalorie) check:** To help prevent yourself from overeating, save some of the calories in your big meal for later. Eat just a portion of your lunch and store it in the fridge for another time. Or when eating out, order just an appetizer and salad and forgo a main course. You can certainly skip dessert, or just eat a piece of fruit instead. Remember, eating small meals throughout the day is better than consuming all your calories in one big meal.

Guidelines for Eating In

Here are some general guidelines for healthy eating, and thus, healthy aging. And, of course, don't forget to eat as many meals as possible from the eight-day meal plan in Part III!

1. **Always eat breakfast:** Be thoughtful about your choices. Your breakfast should represent approximately one-quarter of your daily calories.

   When cooking breakfast, use the oils already mentioned. Organic canola oil is a good choice for eggs and can be sprayed with a mister onto a frying pan to conserve calories. Butter, high in saturated fat, should be used sparingly.

   Make sure that you're giving yourself enough time to eat so you can chew well. Too often breakfast is gulped down on the run, so sit, feel calm, and breathe. If you're feeling stressed at breakfast, you may have had too much caffeine; consider cutting down if you're edgy or anxious.

   Inject some variety into your morning. You don't have to eat cornflakes with skim milk every day. In fact, if you're having cereal, avoid all the highly processed ones and instead pick a high-fiber cereal such as Uncle Sam, Ezekiel 4:9 sprouted cereals, Fiber One, or one of the many other organic, high-fiber brands. You could also try some whole steel-cut oats with a cup of blueberries and a piece of whole-grain toast topped with a little smoked salmon, along with a glass of orange juice.

   Some other good choices: Since you should be eating eight to ten servings of fruits and vegetables during the day, try to get at least three of these servings at breakfast. Don't forget that there are more interesting ways to get your fruits and vegetables than steaming some broccoli. Salsa, which tastes terrific on an omelet, is a great option. Or place a few leftover vegetables in your omelet. Munch on prunes or dried fruit; even the raisins in your raisin bran cereal count as one-half a fruit serving.

2. **Try a midmorning snack:** Instead of relying on the office vending machine for a chocolate bar or a high-fat, overly processed granola bar, bring in a healthy snack from home—a piece of fruit, granola mixed with some nuts and raisins, or

the organic vegetables that now come prewashed in their own small packets.

3. **Plan for lunchtime:** You should be thinking about lunch three or four hours following breakfast.

Not everyone can eat a good lunch at work. But if you know that there are no opportunities to buy healthy foods nearby, prepare something, just as you did for your midmorning snack. Pack a couple pieces of fresh or dried fruit or a small packet of nuts. You can also add a few more of those organic baby carrots or snap peas. Try some fresh berries added to nonfat yogurt (unsweetened has fewer calories), or a small tub of hummus, for dipping those baby carrots. Think about spinach on your sandwich instead of plain iceberg lettuce, and don't forget the tomatoes, onions, and the whole-grain, high-fiber bread.

4. **Eat a midday snack:** Around 3:00 or 4:00 you'll be ready for a quick snack. This is a good time for a hot fudge sundae or a couple of cupcakes—just kidding! But I know you're tired of carrots and peas by now, so how about something different? Among my favorite snacks are Organic Just Fruit and Just Vegetable Munchies made by Just Tomatoes, Etc.! These crunchy, delicious dried fruit and veggie treats come in many varieties and are relatively inexpensive. They're so good you may feel a little guilty. Another excellent choice is a snack bar from a company called Lärabar; containing raw, unprocessed foods, these come in flavors like chocolate coconut and cherry pie and taste almost as good as the real thing.

5. **Give dinner its due:** Dinner is worth planning and preparing for, then savoring fully.

First, consider inviting somebody over, or joining a friend or loved one. You will eat more slowly, and enjoy it more, if you're not rushing through it by yourself. Not that a dinner eaten alone can't be healthy too; it's just that most of us need a companion if we're to eat slowly and carefully. When we're alone, we tend to gulp down the food.

If you're dining at home, play some soothing background music. Light a candle or two. Enjoy a small glass of wine if you are so inclined.

You should have at least two or three servings of steamed, lightly sautéed, or broiled vegetables. Splurge on asparagus, summer squash, steamed spinach, or artichoke.

Be sure to eat fish at least twice a week, and as mentioned, choose smaller fish over tuna steaks or swordfish. When eating meat, lean is your best option; skinless chicken and turkey, game meats, and lean cuts of beef are all acceptable. Trim the (saturated) animal fat.

If you want a dessert, consider fruit. If you absolutely must have something sweeter, have a cookie—but not three or six. Everyone needs to indulge now and then, but never to excess.

The time between dinner and bedtime often challenges people trying to control their eating. Here are some tips to avoid giving in to temptation: Take a walk. Have a cup of hot tea. Snuggle with a loved one. Call a friend on the phone. Go see or rent a movie. Drink a glass of water with a slice of lemon. Get a massage. Give a massage. Do something, anything, besides obsessing about food.

GUIDELINES FOR EATING OUT

Eating well outside the home is one of the biggest challenges to maintaining a healthy immune system. Your favorite restaurant's goal isn't to keep your immune system happy; it's to make your stomach feel satisfied. So restaurant portions are usually gigantic. In fact, over the past twenty years, portion sizes and calorie content of nearly

---

CALORIE COUNTING

Throughout your day, think about your calorie intake as you make food choices.

To roughly calculate your caloric needs to maintain a good, healthy weight, multiply your desired weight by eleven. For instance, if you'd like to weigh 150 pounds, you should be eating about 1,650 calories a day.

To achieve this goal, eat no more than a third of your calories at any one meal, meaning your largest meal should contain about 550 calories. This practice spreads your calories out over the day, and usually allows for two snacks as well.

Two excellent references to calorie counting are Dr. Howard Shapiro's *Picture Perfect Weight Loss,* and Corrine Netzer's *The Complete Book of Food Counts.* Both guides help to give a clear and accurate sense of how many calories you're eating.

---

every type of food served in restaurants have increased dramatically. According to the U.S. Department of Agriculture, bagels are 195 percent larger; steaks, 224 percent larger; muffins, 333 percent larger; pasta entrées, 480 percent larger; and cookies, 700 percent larger.

To hold all this food, the average plate size in restaurants has increased from ten to twelve inches. That means more food, more calories, and more trouble for the immune system. To make matters worse, most restaurants want to maximize the taste of their food, so they load it up with butter, fat, salt, monosodium glutamate, sugar, and/or refined flour.

If you're going to eat out, consider having an appetizer at home so you're less hungry when you arrive at your destination, where you may have to wait some time before ordering and eating. Try salad, chicken satay, or raw vegetables and dip in your own kitchen.

Once at the restaurant, ordering and eating right are a matter of both quantity and quality. Here are some tips to keep in mind.

1. **Don't munch on the bread:** A roll before dinner can represent up to a fifth of the calories for the entire meal; two rolls will total nearly half, especially if you've added butter or oil.

2. **Speak up:** You're paying the restaurant, not vice versa, so don't be shy. Specify exactly how you'd like your food cooked. If chefs hear that patrons prefer healthy food over unhealthy, they may change their methods and menus.

   Ask your server, "How is this dish prepared?" If the answer is that it's breaded, fried, cooked in oil, or sautéed in butter, ask if it can be cooked differently. You'd be amazed at how flexible restaurants can be, especially when you request that they prepare something using less expensive ingredients (saving them, say, a pound of butter in your steamed rather than butter-broiled fish).

3. **Skip the appetizer:** In most restaurants, ordering a soup, salad, and entrée will almost surely produce too much food and too many calories. Skip the appetizer, or consider ordering just the appetizer and a salad.

4. **Stick with salad:** If you're particularly hungry, order a large salad of greens (without the blue cheese, candied walnuts, or butter-soaked croutons) and ask for the dressing on the side. Drizzling dressing results in far fewer calories.

5. **Be wary of fats and oils:** These are the highest in calories of all foods. Salad dressings, olive oil, sautéed or fried foods, fatty meats (including the skin on poultry), and butter all must be eaten sparingly. They can easily put you over your calorie limit

for the day. (Yes, oils such as olive and canola can be good for you and your immune system, but only in moderation—sometimes restaurant salads seem to contain more oil than lettuce.)

6. **Choose lean protein:** Choose lean meats instead of fatty, marbled cuts, and be sure to trim off the visible fat.

7. **Order a veggie side:** An extra side order of veggies will help fill you up and add great immune-friendly nutrients without adding many calories. Good choices include edamame, green beans, peas (any kind), asparagus, cauliflower, and spinach. (But don't let the restaurant use lots of oil or butter to prepare them; steaming is an excellent way to enjoy fresh veggies—it preserves the natural flavor and keeps the vitamins intact.)

8. **Don't clean your plate:** Remember, you don't have to eat everything on your plate! Follow the CHECK List when you're eating out. If you reach the point of feeling full and satisfied, wrap up the rest! It will make a good lunch tomorrow.

9. **Go easy on desserts:** As good as it sounds, it's unlikely to help your immune system, unless it's fruit. But if you really need a sugary dessert, order one dessert for the table and just take a bite. Or try a low-fat decaf cappuccino.

10. **Take your time:** Remember to eat slowly and savor each bite. Put down your utensils after each mouthful and rest your hands in your lap. See if you can become the slowest eater at the table.

STEP 3: SLEEP

RECENTLY A POLITICIAN was discussing his heartbreaking loss in a close election. When a reporter asked him how he felt, he replied: "It really didn't bother me that much. In fact, the night I lost the election, I slept like a baby—I slept two hours, then I woke up crying. I slept two more hours, and I woke up crying."

That's what sleep means for many of us, much of the time—a dizzying combination of actual sleeping amid cycles of waking, dreaming, thinking, worrying, and so on. Yet a good night's sleep is one of the most important means at our disposal to calm our immune system.

Remember that the immune system resembles a second brain. It tracks your emotions just as the mind does. It knows when you're worried, threatened, or upset just as your mind senses these emotions. It hears the same signals.

One of the most important cues the immune system listens to is sleep. Yet just as we take breathing for granted, we often take sleep for granted. We do this because we begin life as excellent sleepers. Children tend to sleep very well, as do teens. Most people have to reach adulthood before they start to appreciate sleep—or the lack thereof.

When I was younger, I worked in an emergency room, where staying up all night was routine. After a shift, I'd go home, kiss my kids as they went off to school, and take a three-hour nap. That was it. Today, I'd need to sleep for eight hours to recover from just one night of that routine, no less several years of it.

These days, adult Americans experience an increasing number of sleep disorders. The causes are numerous.

Perhaps the most obvious is that people are growing increasingly stressed. With every passing year, the modern world seems more and more complicated, as does our ability to compete in our ever-changing, ever-more-difficult culture. Even the world itself seems more threatening. Many patients tell me that they can't sleep because they've been spending so much time reading the bad news from all over the globe, from famine to war, from crime to climatological disaster. There's no shortage of worrisome events, and these weigh heavily on sleep quality.

Another reason people aren't sleeping well is substance abuse. By that I don't mean hard drugs; I mean caffeine. Today it seems as if there's a coffee bar on every corner of every city; there are currently more than 150 Starbucks locations in Manhattan alone.

The problem with caffeine is that its half-life is more than six hours, which means that six hours after you've drunk your last cup of coffee, half the caffeine remains in your system; six hours after that, a quarter is still left. Certain conditions, such as pregnancy, prolong that half-life even further, extending it to as much as eighteen hours; taking birth control pills extends the half-life of caffeine to more than twelve hours. Many medications prolong caffeine's half-life as well, including the antibiotics Cipro and Levaquin, the antacid Tagamet, the antidepressant Luvox, the asthma medicine Zyflo, and the HIV drug Reyataz, to name just a few. Even grapefruit juice and green tea significantly prolong the effects of caffeine in the body.

So it's easy to see that when people need to wind down, they're often too caffeinated to manage it. What do they do? Many end up drinking alcohol to numb themselves into a sleepy stupor. All they're really doing is temporarily numbing their brain cells. Drinking alcohol may enable you to fall asleep, but your liver will immediately start processing the alcohol, and three or four hours later, your blood alcohol levels will return to nearly zero. Now you'll begin to experience a mini withdrawal syndrome that's very stimulating. In fact, it causes arousal—and you'll wake up.

Yawn! You've created a vicious circle that, over time, leads to sleep deprivation.

Caffeine and alcohol aren't the only things that hinder sleep. There's also the widespread use of sleep medications. Sleeping pills now rank among the most highly prescribed medications. The problem with such medications is that, while they can indeed help you fall asleep, they won't keep you asleep. When the pills wear off a few hours after you take them, you may well wake up again and find yourself unable to get back to sleep. You may then be tempted to take another pill.

Sleeping pills can be habit-forming and even addictive. When you take such pills for more than a few days in a row, you build up a tolerance and may find that you need a higher and higher dose to fall asleep. As the dose escalates, you may fall into addiction.

Perhaps these reasons for lack of sleep aren't a surprise—but did you know that excess weight can also affect sleep? The recent obesity epidemic has taken its toll on sleep as well as on health, because overweight people have more difficulty sleeping than others. For one thing, they can't find a comfortable position in bed: if they lie on their back, they can't breathe well; if they lie on their stomach, their breathing can become even more restricted. They end up constantly tired, and no matter how much time they spend in bed, they never seem to catch up on their rest. That fatigue only causes them to need even more time in bed.

THE IMPORTANCE OF HIGH-QUALITY SLEEP

Few issues concern patients as much as sleep. "How can I get more?" is probably the most common question I hear.

The real issue, however, is not the quantity of sleep; it's the quality. Five hours of good sleep can be as refreshing as seven hours of bad sleep.

Scientists have recognized five stages of sleep, which are divided into two basic types—REM (rapid eye movement) and non-REM sleep.

REM sleep usually represents about 25 percent of the time spent sleeping. Dreaming takes place during this stage.

Non-REM sleep has four stages, each of which is progressively deeper. Stages III and IV are generally considered deep sleep, while stage IV in particular is the recuperative sleep that restores and recharges your body.

During each night, our sleep cycles through all the different stages. It's normal to experience periods of light sleep (stages I and II) interspersed with deep sleep (stages III and IV) and dreaming (REM sleep). As the night progresses, we tend to have more frequent REM sleep, and in the early morning most of our sleep is REM—which explains, in part, why we often remember our dreams as we awaken.

Scientists don't understand exactly what takes place inside our brains, or our bodies, during the different stages of non-REM and REM sleep, but a few concepts seem clear. For the most part, during REM sleep you are lying very still, and even though your eyes are moving rapidly, your arms and legs are completely motionless. This stillness explains why you may sometimes awake with lines on your face, or with tingling arms, from the uncomfortable positions you fall into—and remain in—during REM sleep.

Brain-wave measurements can help us to understand some of the brain activity that occurs during different phases of sleep.

Deep sleep (stages III and IV) ushers in the appearance of so-called delta waves on the brain-wave, or EEG, measurement. These slow waves represent the most restorative sleep. In contrast, during REM sleep, brain waves show a fairly active pattern that includes beta waves, which are also present during active thinking.

A lack of deep, restorative sleep, or of delta waves, has been repeatedly shown to cause immune activation. Consider sleep apnea; sufferers endure frequent and repeated episodes of halted breathing during sleep. This cessation often occurs because the person's airway closes off, due to, for example, sleeping position; it's most prevalent when people lie on their back. However, sleep apnea most frequently results from being overweight, because of the added thickness of the neck, cheeks, and tongue.

Whatever its cause, the restricted airway triggers a blockage of airflow, just as if you had held your breath purposefully.

When you consciously hold your breath, your carbon dioxide level starts to climb. Then you feel uncomfortable. Your heart rate increases. Now you desperately want to take a breath, you become very agitated, and eventually you just have to breathe—and you do.

That same process occurs in people with sleep apnea—their brain, recognizing they're not breathing, sends a signal to arouse them. They then become restless, move around, and, usually with a loud snort, begin to breathe again. This arousal wakes them just enough to yank them out of deep sleep but not enough to wake them fully.

The problem here is that if apnea occurs too often, sufferers don't spend sufficient time in restorative sleep. Their brain will keep rousing them to restore their breathing, and they have to start the sleep cycle all over again at stage I. (Unfortunately, you can't arrive at stage IV without going through the first three stages.)

The result: people with sleep apnea never receive enough restorative deep sleep. So they never get their metaphorical batteries recharged, even if they stay in bed for nine hours. They always feel tired. They're always dragging. They need to take naps and go to bed early.

Recent research has shown that sleep apnea sufferers also have higher levels of immune activation and higher CRP levels than normal sleepers. Studies from the Mayo Clinic, published in *Circulation* in May 2002, showed that patients with sleep apnea have CRP levels almost four times higher than those without. Research from Penn State University published in the *Journal of Clinical Endocrinology & Metabolism* in February 1997 also showed elevated levels of the cytokines interleukin-6 and TNF-alpha in patients with sleep apnea. Successful treatment of sleep apnea and the resumption of quality, deep sleep resulted in lowering of the subjects' CRP and cytokine levels.

THE IMMUNE SYSTEM AND SLEEP

I said earlier that it's the quality, not the quantity, of sleep that counts. Some people need to be in bed for seven hours, some for five, others for nine. The differences in quantity of sleep required probably are due to the quality of that sleep.

Unfortunately, it's very difficult to measure this quality. Unless somebody attaches electrodes to your head and prints out a brain-wave map, you can't know for sure how much high-quality sleep you're getting.

Your behavioral patterns during the day can provide useful clues, however. For example, do you often fall asleep while you're reading a book or watching TV? Do you ever start to nod off when you're driving your car for more than an hour or two? Do you doze in church? Do you find that you have to catch up on your sleep during the weekends? Do you wake up most mornings feeling tired rather than rested?

If so, you're not getting enough quality sleep. You might be getting quantity sleep because you go to bed at, say, 10:30 p.m. and rise at 7 a.m. But if you're still waking up tired, or feeling any of the above symptoms, you're probably not sleeping well.

Research shows that the immune system exerts a powerful effect on sleep. For reasons that aren't yet completely understood, there are times when our immune system plays a key role in regulating our sleep.

Immune system cytokines, including interleukins and TNF-alpha, affect the quality and stages of our sleep. All of us have had the flu or a bad cold or some other type of infection. When we're sick, we want to sleep all day, and even after we've woken up, we're still drowsy. It's these cytokines, produced by the immune system, that make us feel this way.

The cytokines increase delta-wave (slow-wave) sleep and reduce REM sleep. When we are trying to recover from an infection, we need more rest, and in this way, our immune system and brain work together to produce more deep sleep.

Immune activation is probably the reason some people often feel lethargic even when they don't have an infection. The lower the levels of immune activation, the more energetic, and less sleepy, you are likely to feel, and vice versa.

(Of course, there is an obvious feedback loop here: if you're not getting enough sleep for whatever reason, you are activating your immune system; the immune system then produces the cytokines that make you sleepy, and so on.)

You may have heard of the disease known as sleeping sickness, which is caused by a parasitic protozoan (single-celled organism) called a trypanosome and is most commonly found in Africa. Symptoms of the disease, as you've probably guessed, are fatigue and sleepiness. The production of cytokines by the immune systems of infected individuals may be contributing to the sleepiness associated with trypanosome infection.

The immune system senses whether or not you have slept well. The better you sleep, the better it functions—ready, willing, and able to respond to any threat, but not overly active. When you're getting enough deep, restful sleep, your immune system is calm and relaxed, and its cytokine production is turned off.

Though I've said quality matters more than quantity when it comes to sleep, getting the right amount of sleep is critical for your immune system; it requires sleep just as much as your brain does.

Brain researchers have found that while you sleep, your brain is repairing itself—something it can't do at any other time. During a normal day, small connections in the brain can break, nutrients become depleted, and infrastructure needs repair; moreover, memory storage needs to be shifted, or "defragmented." All of these small problems need to be remedied, and the brain knows how to do that—when it's turned off.

It's not unlike your computer. When major repairs are required, you don't do them while the computer is up and running; repairs take place while the computer is down. Likewise, your brain can't repair itself while it's thinking, looking about, finding something to eat, and so on. Your brain's too busy making sure you survive.

Like the brain, the immune system is constantly busy during the day: storing memories; examining every bit of food that you've digested; trying to figure out if there's a friend or foe coming along; and communicating, as each and every cell talks to all the other cells throughout the body and tells them what it bumped into that day, shares memories, produces antibodies, and plays its part in taking care of your health. The immune system relies on sleep for a chance to repair, recharge, and perform its maintenance functions on your body.

Also, the immune system requires that our stress levels be turned off at regular intervals. Simply being awake and functioning during the day is a stressful process. Your immune system must remain constantly on alert, because anything can happen: a bicyclist could crash into you, your boss could yell at you, a bacterium or a grizzly bear could attack you.

During sleep, however, your stress levels are sufficiently diminished so the immune system can recharge. But if, as you sleep, you're feeling stress, the immune system can't relax. For example, night terrors can cause your immune system to become overactive; these terrors are recognized as a sleep disorder that occurs during non-REM sleep, and they are one of the symptoms of sleep apnea.

Researchers conjecture that they could, in part, result from the failure to breathe well, which in turn causes high levels of immune activation.

In the sleep disorder narcolepsy, people can be in the middle of a conversation when they abruptly fall asleep. Researchers at the Stanford Center for Narcolepsy Research found significantly elevated levels of the cytokines interleukin-1 and TNF-alpha in the blood of narcoleptic patients, indicating immune activation and elevated cytokines (*Brain, Behavior, and Immunity*, July 2004).

INSOMNIA

Just as sleep apnea and narcolepsy activate the immune system, so does insomnia.

Insomnia has a number of different causes. One is self-imposed, by people who don't allot themselves enough time to sleep, or have unusual sleep arrangements.

Another type of insomnia is caused by mood disorders such as anxiety and depression. Sufferers don't sleep well because they're too worried—perhaps they're going through a divorce, or have sick loved ones, or they're caretakers who are always listening for a partner to fall out of bed, or an alarm, or the sound of a baby's cry.

Research in 2003 conducted at Harvard Medical School and the Brigham and Women's Hospital studied the effects of insomnia on immune activation and CRP levels. In the study, researchers kept ten healthy adults awake for eighty-eight straight hours. The subjects' CRP levels were tested every ninety minutes for five days; over this period, the volunteers' levels rose to about five times the normal amount.

In a second experiment, ten volunteers were allowed to sleep only 4.2 hours each night for ten consecutive nights. Hourly CRP levels were measured, and again CRP levels rose about fivefold.

In a study of more than twenty-eight thousand children and fifteen thousand adults, researchers at England's Warwick Medical School found that shorter sleep duration was linked with almost double the normal risk of obesity, and that this risk held even for children as young as five years old.

And findings from the Nurses Health Study, involving 71,617 female nurses, revealed that women who slept five hours or less per night were 45 percent more likely to suffer heart problems. Even sleeping six hours a night was linked with a nearly 20 percent increase in heart problems.

Sleep deprivation and insomnia are important causes of immune activation. Thus it's little surprise that sleep deprivation has been shown to not only double the risk of obesity but to increase the risk of heart disease as well.

Good quality sleep is important for health, for the immune system, and to decelerate aging. Impairment from sleep deprivation is equivalent to that from alcohol intoxication. When asked to perform various tasks, from simple calculations to walking a line, people who are sleep-deprived perform just as badly as those who are legally intoxicated.

The familiar concepts of getting one's beauty sleep or sleeping like a baby are age-old and widespread—with good reason. If you're not sleeping well, you're not aging well.

TAKE ACTION: SLEEP

Sleep is very much a habit. It is also a learned behavior. This means you can retrain your mind and body to get back into the habit of sleeping well. But it takes practice.

Sleep conditioning is most successful if you follow these steps consistently. If you're training dogs, for example, you don't let them jump on the couch "sometimes." They shouldn't be taught to come "now and then." You need to be consistent to produce the desired behavior.

An erratic sleeping pattern may suffice for those who have no trouble falling asleep. However, such people are rare. The rest of us must do everything possible to get a good night's rest. Besides steady habits, that means creating the right environment and mastering the ability to relax the mind and body.

By following the guidelines outlined here, you're most likely to succeed.

THE DOS

1. **Set a bedtime:** Sleep should have a uniform pattern. In other words, you should try to go to sleep at the same time every night and wake up at the same time every morning. Humans weren't meant to go to bed at 9 p.m. one night, stay up until 2 a.m. the next, then go to sleep at 8 p.m. the following night. The body can't learn to settle into the right habits with an erratic sleep pattern.

   Set a bedtime. It doesn't matter whether you choose 10 p.m. or 1 a.m. as long as you stick to it. Some people are morning people—they want to get up at 5 a.m. and watch the sunrise. Others want to sleep until 10 a.m. or later. That's fine too. But it's a mistake to alter the pattern, even on weekends, when you might want to sleep in. (If you're finding that you always need to sleep in on the weekends, you're probably not giving yourself enough quality sleep during the week.)

   The Eastern health discipline known as Ayurveda recognizes and values the timing of cycles during the day. According to the practice, cycles progress in six four-hour units, beginning with awakening at 6 a.m. and with bedtime ideally set at

10 p.m. This pattern allows for eight hours of sleep and is said to be harmonious with the activity of the human mind and body.

If you're following this pattern properly, you won't need an alarm clock, because you'll find you always awaken naturally at the same time.

2. **Create a peaceful sleep environment:** Allow as few distractions as possible. No noise, light, television, computers, or pagers should be present.

   Most important: darkness. Your clock shouldn't be glowing, light shouldn't be shining under your door, the moon—or streetlights—shouldn't be glowing through your windows.

   Some people create a calming sleep environment by lighting candles in their bedroom, so that when they're ready for sleep, they walk into a soothing setting. (Remember to blow them out before sleeping, however; flickering lights aren't helpful or safe.)

   You'll want an inviting bed environment as well: a restful mattress, soft sheets, cozy blankets, and comfortable pillows, so that when you slip into bed, you say, "Ahhhh!" If your sheets are scratchy, your bedclothes messy, and the mattress lumpy, you simply won't sleep well.

3. **Develop a sleep ritual:** A sleep ritual creates a conditioned response in which your body, your brain, and your immune system experience a familiar pattern that automatically leads to sleep.

   For example, some people like to read in bed for half an hour. Others use a relaxation process, such as meditation, breathing exercises, or a few simple yoga poses. Still others like to write down all the things they have to worry about the next day, so they won't obsess about them before, and while, they sleep.

Another sleep-conditioning technique is a muscle-relaxation exercise in which you relax one muscle at a time throughout your body, moving from your toes up to your feet, ankles, calves, knees, thighs, hips, back, belly, shoulders, arms, fingers, neck, and finally your face. By the time your face is completely relaxed—along with the rest of your body—you should be able to fall asleep.

And, of course, some people count sheep, or count backwards from one hundred.

Here's a simple meditation exercise that can help bring on sleep. First, sit next to your bed (a chair or a pillow on the floor is equally fine, but leave the bed itself for sleeping only). Try to keep your back straight. Close your eyes. Take in three deep breaths, each time exhaling completely. Concentrate on your slow breathing, and with each breath out, feel the stress and tension leave your body. Now focus your mind on one thing that you love dearly, whether it's a mate, child, friend, pet, or even an activity or object. Center on its essence. Feel all other thoughts, concerns, and tensions leave your mind. Sense your mind calming and your body feeling lighter. Continue your slow breathing, exhaling fully with each breath. If your mind wanders, don't be upset; just calmly regain your focus.

Continue this meditation until you feel completely relaxed and calm and all the tension has drained from your body. At this point, move to your bed and fall into a gentle, deep slumber.

4. **Find appropriate sleep accessories:** Don't worry about what you look like while you sleep. If you need help keeping light out, buy a cloth eyeshade. They come in various types and sizes, and work especially well for people whose bedrooms let in light no matter how many curtains and window shades have been hung.

   Similarly, some people's bedrooms are noisy. If this is the

case for you, get earplugs. They come in many different varieties and materials. Inexpensive foam earplugs work quite well, and they're usually comfortable even for people who sleep on their side. These plugs may take some getting used to, but I've never run into anyone who couldn't find a pair that felt comfortable enough to ensure a good night's sleep.

Also, if you enjoy sleeping in pajamas, splurge a little and find a few pairs that are unrestricting, soft, and comforting. Flannels in the winter and cotton or silk in warmer weather work well.

5. **Talk to your sleep partner:** If you sleep with someone, ask him or her to help you. If something is bothering you, get it off your chest. Allow your partner to soothe you. Snuggle. Make love. Massage each other's neck, shoulders, or feet. A scalp massage is especially relaxing and easy to do. A foot massage, using a bit of massage oil, is also tremendously relaxing.

Talk with your partner about other ways you can help each other to sleep better. It's important for him or her to learn how best to work with you, particularly if he or she is doing something that's keeping you awake. These discussions can be helpful in making adjustments to sleep positions, and deciding what to do if your partner wakes up often, frequently gets out of bed, or snores.

For some people, sleeping with a pet can be soothing. But as much as you may love your animal companions, if they are depriving you of sleep, consider keeping them off the bed—or out of the bedroom altogether if they wake you up every morning begging for love, or breakfast.

6. **Use your nose:** Certain aromas may help you sleep—aromatherapeutic oils can have a soothing effect on the body.

Although tastes vary from person to person, some oils that seem effective include jasmine, geranium, rose, and marjoram. You can place five to eight drops in a presleep bath, or buy an aromatic diffuser and let the odor waft through the room. You can also put a drop on a handkerchief and place it inside your pillowcase before you sleep.

7. **Take a bath:** A soothing, hot bath, infused with essential oils and taken before going to sleep, can help rest both body and mind, easing and relaxing sore muscles. It will also help calm your thoughts and your breathing. Inhaling the humidified air evaporating from a hot bath helps to hydrate and soothe the lungs and airways.

   If you feel a little achy, add one-half cup Epsom salts (magnesium sulfate) to the water, plus an equal measure of baking soda (sodium bicarbonate).

8. **Develop a dream mantra:** A mantra is a mental pattern on which to focus. Try conjuring one up before going to bed. A mantra doesn't have to be verbal. You can use an image, a thought, or a feeling. But your mind quiets down when you can lead it to focus on just one thing.

   I know some people who like the phrase "I am so happy to be in bed," and others who create a lovely image of a place where no one can bother them, or who conjure up a happy memory from the past. A mantra can be the mental image of swinging in a hammock in a grass-roofed hut, or lying with a lover, or floating in the ocean.

   If you can create a successful dream mantra, eventually other intrusive thoughts will dissipate and you can drift into sleep. With practice, some people get so good that they can fall asleep almost immediately after conjuring up their dream mantra.

The Don'ts

1. **Don't overcaffeinate:** Pay attention to the quantity of stimulants, including caffeinated sodas and chocolate, that you ingest during the day. As mentioned, caffeine taken in the afternoon has effects at bedtime. Restrict your caffeine to mornings only.

   Alcohol is also a stimulant, so if you find you are waking up a few hours after going to sleep, steer clear of alcohol—even that glass of wine with dinner.

2. **Don't overstimulate:** Avoid watching the news on TV, surfing Internet news sites, or answering work-related e-mails before bed. Disturbing images and current events, or troublesome e-mails from work, will keep your mind churning and make it much more difficult to fall asleep.

3. **Don't overdo nighttime liquid intake:** The urge to urinate is a common reason to awaken during the night. If you're going too often, try reducing fluid intake two hours before bedtime—and don't forget to empty your bladder just before bed.

4. **Don't eat before sleep:** It takes a couple of hours to digest food, and it's a process that works best when you are upright, not lying down in bed. Furthermore, this is not the best time to be adding calories to your system. Instead of snacking, if you feel restless, try a soothing bath, or lighting some candles, or meditating. A cup of chamomile tea is fine, as long as your bladder is not already waking you up at night.

5. **Don't use your bed for anything but sleeping (and lovemaking):** If you use your bed as a place to answer e-mails, watch TV, or talk on the phone, you're sending the wrong message to your brain. Your goal is to retrain your body to sleep easily

and deeply. That training requires a consistent message—that bed is for sleeping, and when you enter it, you're ready for rest, not work.

6. **Don't go to bed angry:** If you're mad at your mate, talk it out. Don't take the issue to bed with you. Lying in bed stewing in your own juices will activate your immune system and prevent you from falling asleep. Make a pact: Don't go to bed mad. Resolve the issue beforehand if it's at all possible.

7. **Don't obsess about sleep:** No one has ever died of insomnia (except in very rare cases involving serious genetic sleep disorders). The more worried you are about it, the tougher it gets. Sleep will come. Be patient. You can learn to do it better. Practice. Practice. Practice. *Shhh.* Soon you'll be fast asleep.

STEP 4: DANCE

WHEN YOU THINK of dance, you might imagine a jitterbug, a salsa, a samba, a fox-trot, a waltz, a tango, or maybe even belly dancing, square dancing, or two-stepping. All of these dances are wonderful. But when we talk about dance in the context of the Ultra-Longevity program, we mean something broader: any combination of rhythm and movement.

Rhythmic movement, or moving to a particular rhythm, is the essence of any dance. So whenever you are moving in rhythm, whether or not music is playing, you can consider yourself to be dancing.

This means there's a whole new world of dance out there: the dance of walking, jogging, biking, swimming, hiking, and even golf—after all, good golfers know that their best swings are made when they are following a rhythm. (Many golf pros recommend counting out a beat, starting on the backswing and continuing through the follow-through. Keeping in rhythm maintains the timing of the swing, shot after shot, so you develop consistency.)

Even tennis is a dance. Anyone who's watched a top tennis match knows the game's rhythm, punctuated by the whoosh, pop, whoosh, pop sounds of the volleys. Even the crowd of spectators develop a rhythm, turning their heads and eyes left, then right, then left, then right—the stadium performing a simple dance in unison.

EXERCISE: THE NUMBER ONE
ANTIAGING MEDICINE

Nearly everyone is aware that movement, or exercise, is beneficial to one's health. (But for reasons to be explained shortly, rhythmic movement turns out to be better for you than movement without rhythm.) The most important new discoveries about movement confirm that it offers benefits across a wide range of health conditions, and has a positive impact on the immune system and on aging itself.

Movement may well be the closest thing to the Fountain of Youth ever studied. Dr. Robert Butler, president of the International Longevity Center at Manhattan's Mount Sinai Hospital, has said that if exercise could be packaged in pill form, it would immediately become the number one antiaging medicine, as well as the world's most prescribed pill. An avid exerciser at seventy-eight years old, Bob Butler, who looks like a man half his age, is a walking testimonial to the health benefits of exercise.

Many other examples demonstrate that exercise can prolong, and even save, lives. Consider my hero, Jack LaLanne, who at the age of ninety-two continues to work out for two hours every day. Jack's daily exercise program includes chin-ups and push-ups, as well as weights. A one-man tour de force, with more energy than most forty-year-olds, Jack has been exercising vigorously for more than seventy years. In fact, he was working out long before it was fashionable, and before the health benefits were as well known. Even at his advanced age, Jack doesn't take any medications, and, knock wood, is never sick. (He does admit to taking forty or fifty supplements a day in addition to eating an all-natural, unprocessed, whole-foods diet.)

Jack's health is no fluke. State-of-the-art scientific research has repeatedly shown us the same thing: regular exercise is critical for maintaining ideal health and slowing the effects of aging.

EXERCISE AND THE IMMUNE SYSTEM

As usual, if it's good for your health, it's good for your immune system. Extensive research links exercise and movement with reduced levels of immune activation and lower levels of cytokines and CRP—and you've already read enough of this book to know how important that is.

For example, an April 2006 study of almost four thousand adults (published in *Atherosclerosis*) found that physical activity and fitness level were also inversely correlated with CRP levels. Interestingly, that effect was independent of obesity—that is, whether or not the study's subjects were overweight, the more physically fit and active they were, the lower their CRP.

Many studies have supported these findings, including a May 2006 report in the *International Journal of Cardiology* from the National Health and Nutrition Examination Survey of 1,438 adults between twenty and forty-nine years old. The conclusion: CRP levels were inversely related to cardiorespiratory fitness.

Another study (*Circulation*, 2002) showed that people who exercised most often had the lowest CRP levels and white blood cell counts. Again, this study showed the effect to be independent of weight.

Similar results have been reported in children. A study of more than two hundred children (published in the February 2003 *Journal of Pediatrics*) revealed that the greater the amount of exercise performed, the lower the CRP levels. This study also examined individuals with various disease conditions, including diabetes and prediabetes, and found that after just four weeks in a physical training program, diabetics and prediabetics achieved near normalization of their CRP levels.

The relationship between aerobic fitness and reduced immune activation appears to hold across gender, age, and body size differences. In a study of nearly one hundred young women in Japan, reported in the April 2006 *Endocrine Journal,* regular exercise significantly reduced levels of immune activation as measured by subjects' CRP, TNF-alpha, and leptin levels, even in overweight and obese women.

The effects of exercise on the immune system have also been studied down to the cellular level, so the precise mechanisms by which exercise affects our white blood cells and other parts of the immune system are becoming clearer.

Immunology researchers from the James H. Quillen College of Medicine at East Tennessee State University examined the effects of exercise on white blood cells themselves. White blood cells are known to play an important role in development of heart disease and atherogenesis—the formation of plaques in the arteries around the heart. Scientists found that exercise had a direct effect on the atherogenic propensity of white blood cells. They measured the production of immune-activating and immune-protective cytokines by white blood cells in study subjects before and after exercise.

After six months of weekly exercise (about two and one-half hours per week), the levels of immune-activating cytokines produced by subjects' white blood cells dropped by more than 58 percent, while their levels of immune-protective cytokines rose by more than 35 percent.

These researchers concluded that exercise directly affects the white blood cells' production of immune-activating and -protective cytokines, and that this mechanism was one of the ways in which exercise protects against heart disease.

In fact, exercise is probably the single most effective way to lower CRP levels. If your CRP level is elevated, starting a regular exercise program will lower it. In a study of 652 sedentary men and women, a twenty-week exercise program consistently and significantly lowered their CRP levels independent of any changes in body weight, cholesterol, or blood sugar levels.

THE POWER OF RHYTHM

When physical activity is done to rhythm, it can be considered dance—and dance is a powerful way to get the most benefit from your exercise program.

There are several reasons why adding rhythm to your movements is better than engaging in more random or inconsistent ones. One is that dancing, rather than just moving, has the greatest effect on CRP levels.

Scientists first began investigating this topic in the 1980s; since then many studies have been published. Among the first was an April 1984 study in the *International Journal of Sports Medicine*, showing that when people moved, but especially when they moved rhythmically, their CRP levels dropped.

The study measured the CRP levels of athletes from various sports to see whose were lowest. The results: those who moved most rhythmically enjoyed the lowest CRP levels. Swimmers had the lowest CRP levels of all; swimming, with its left, right, left, right stroking and kicking, is among the most rhythmic of exercises. The second-lowest levels were found in rowers, who also engage in a rhythmic process—they even have a coxswain in the boat to call out the beat. Soccer players' levels were not as low, despite the level of exertion required during a match—there is much less rhythm involved in running and kicking a soccer ball than in swimming or rowing.

A meta-analysis of a group of studies, published in the July/ August 2004 Polish psychology journal *Psychiatry*, reported the effects of exercise on anxiety and depression. Researchers confirmed the benefit of moderate- and low-intensity exercise on mood, and found that this benefit was most pronounced in people who performed rhythmic exercises such as jogging, swimming, cycling, and walking.

Research on healing in rats after spinal cord injury, reported in the journal *Brain* (June 2004), found that rhythmic, weight-bearing exercise was most effective in promoting the rodents' recovery.

Adding music to the rehabilitation and physical therapy programs of Parkinson's disease patients has also been shown to improve outcome when compared with standard physical therapy (*Psychosomatic Medicine,* May/June 2000). Participants receiving music therapy also scored higher on a happiness measure.

Adding rhythm to movement certainly increases the level of enjoyment and involvement in exercise classes. As most health clubs have recognized, the addition of pumping, rhythmic music to aerobic exercise classes encourages participation and increases satisfaction levels.

The explosive growth and popularity of the iPod among exercisers is little surprise. Turning a standard exercise routine into a dance is more fun, less boring, and ensures that exercisers keep at their activity longer.

OUR BUILT-IN RHYTHMS

Several theories exist as to why rhythm is such an important component of movement.

Our muscles come in pairs—one muscle flexes a joint, the other extends it. For example, our quadriceps (thigh) muscles extend our knee, while the hamstrings flex it. Rhythmic contraction, alternating between flexion and extension, provides balance, and strengthens both flexors and extensors equally.

The nerve impulses that regulate paired muscle groups originate from signals in our brain and are transmitted along the spinal cord. Rhythmic movement creates a pattern in the brain and spinal cord that is also transmitted to our immune system—the same neurotransmitter chemicals released by our brain and nerve endings are sensed by our immune system. When our brain is dancing, so is our immune system.

While scientists can't yet explain fully why this link to rhythm in exercise is so important, it certainly appeals to common sense. Consider the many intrinsic rhythms built into the living, breathing human body.

As discussed, our breath is always rhythmic—when we're breathing well, we're breathing rhythmically. Disruptions in our breathing rhythm, usually an ominous sign, are highly activating to the immune system.

Or consider the body's most obvious rhythm: the heartbeat. Loss of the normal heart rhythm has also been linked with immune activation. A common heart arrhythmia is known as atrial fibrillation; CRP levels are elevated in people who develop this condition. CRP has also been found to be elevated in more serious, even lethal, arrhythmias of the heart, including ventricular fibrillation and sudden cardiac death. It's vital to our immune health that our heart maintain its regular rhythm.

Several other body rhythms are less obvious, such as peristalsis of the gut, during which a rhythmic wave alternately contracts and relaxes, starting far up in the stomach and ending far down in the colon, to move food from north to south. Brain waves are also rhythmic. So are circadian (or daily) biorhythms, women's menstrual cycles, and the rhythmic contractions of the uterus during labor. Our glands release hormones in rhythmic patterns, such as the pulsating release of growth hormones from the pituitary gland and the gradual release of melatonin from our pineal glands. And, of course, sexual intercourse is exquisitely rhythmic in nature.

The immune system actually has its own circadian rhythm that seems to be linked with our cycle of sleep and wakefulness.

In so many ways, human life itself consists of rhythms; it's quite possible the immune system responds to these rhythms. There's even a new type of medical treatment called chronotherapy that uses this effect to advantage by timing the application of certain therapies. Timing has a tangible impact on the outcome of such treatments.

For example, asthma attacks tend to occur in the early morning hours. That's often the time when a sufferer's asthma medicine has worn off, especially if the most recent dose was taken the previous evening. Thus new delayed-release medications have been developed; these are taken at night but don't start working until they're needed most, in the early morning.

A similar pattern occurs with blood pressure, which peaks in the early morning, around 7 or 8 a.m., often before people have taken their first dose of blood pressure medication, leaving a window when the patient is not protected. Unremediated early morning high blood pressure is one explanation for why more heart attacks occur in the morning than at other times. And here, too, new delayed-release medications can help offset the danger.

Chronotherapy is also used in cancer treatment with chemotherapy. Chemotherapy works primarily by targeting cell division, killing rapidly dividing cancer cells. Many of chemotherapy's side effects result from the fact that some normal cells are also killed as they divide. These side effects can include damage to the mucous membranes (e.g., the lining of the mouth, esophagus, and intestinal tract) or harm to the white blood cells themselves, which are formed from stem cells dividing in the bone marrow.

Chronotherapy takes advantage of the timing of normal cell division by providing chemotherapy during times when the process is less active. This treatment has been found to reduce chemotherapy's side effects, while allowing the dose to be increased and, therefore, more effective in killing the medicine's targets—cancer cells.

Scientists are learning how to use new information about the body's natural rhythms to make other therapies more effective, reduce side effects, and more precisely target the offending cells or germs. The more we learn about the body's natural rhythms, the more likely we are to develop effective therapies that work with the body rather than against it.

THE DANCE OF LIFE

The research on rhythm and dance as an essential part of life and health is new, but the concept of rhythm as an integral part of life is as old as history.

In the most ancient of all religions, Hinduism, dancing is thought to be the origin of the universe. Shiva, one of the three gods of the Hindu trinity that also includes Brahma and Vishnu, emanates the entire universe through what's known as the cosmic dance of Shiva.

Observation confirms the infinite variety of rhythms in the universe—the sunrise and sunset, the changing of the seasons, the rotation and orbits of the planets, the ebb and flow of the tides, the waxing and waning of the moon, the flapping of a bird's wings, the buzzing of a bee, or the suckling of an infant. In Hinduism, the frequency and rhythm of all such sounds are considered to hold healing powers, as in the vocalization *om* ("ah-ooh-mm") and in the many healing mantras recited in Eastern religions.

Rhythm and dance also abound in Greek mythology. Apollo, the son of Zeus and the god of medicine, was known as the dancer—already a connection was being made between dance and health. In Sparta, one of ancient Greece's most powerful city-states, authorities required parents to instruct their children in the art of dancing, beginning at the age of five. Dancing was thought to be good for the body and overall health, as well as for the soul.

Moving to modern science, research has shown that music and rhythm produce measurable healing effects. Music has been proven to reduce stress and anxiety, as evidenced by multiple studies of heart patients who underwent catheterization tests, an unpleasant procedure in which a tube is inserted in the heart. These patients' anxiety levels were significantly reduced when music was played during cardiac catheterization (*Clinical Research in Cardiology,* August 2006).

Music can even lessen pain, as shown by a Korean study in which music therapy was found to reduce the pain of fractures in people with broken legs. Similarly, music reduced agitation and anxiety in patients with Alzheimer's disease (*International Psychogeriatrics,* April 2006).

Studies also reveal that our brain uses rhythm to heal. Researchers at the Helen Willis Neuroscience Center at the University of California, Berkeley, reported in *Science* (September 15, 2006) that rhythmic discharges of neurons in the brain encourage brain healing and repair. So-called theta rhythms are slow, rhythmic brain waves that, for reasons not yet understood, are an important part of plasticity, or the healing of synapses between brain nerves.

Being out of rhythm with the body is often linked with immune activation. We've talked about the importance of breathing well, and how, when our breath is out of rhythm, immune activation results. Similarly, when the heartbeat is irregular, we also see immune activation, as we do when menstrual cycles or even bowel habits are irregular.

In contrast, the benefits of rhythm plus movement (or dance in any form) seem endless. Dance improves everything from our balance and gait to bone density in the legs and hips. It creates a better mood. It's been shown to help with weight loss and to improve cardiovascular fitness. It lowers cholesterol levels.

Perhaps one of the reasons movement and rhythm are such a powerful combination is that together they create something of a trance state.

Healers across many different cultures have employed dance to induce a trance as part of a healing ritual. In southern Italy, for example, the *pizzica tarantata* was a therapeutic dance performed to heal the bite of the tarantula. Many Native American cultures, including the Apache, Sioux, and Cree, used medicine dances as healing rituals. The !Kung tribe of the Kalahari desert in Africa practices the "giraffe dance" as a healing art; dancers and singers intensify their trancelike dance until healers reach a state of altered consciousness, at which point they focus their energies toward healing the community's ill.

The Chinese discipline known as tai chi, which originated more than eight centuries ago, is still widely used as a healing art. Using a dancelike movement and inducing a trance, tai chi creates a meditative state that is said to restore natural rhythms and balance in the mind and body.

The hypnotic state sought through ancient dance rituals has two basic qualities. One is a dissociation from the normal physical environment; you're not as distracted by external events. The other is a narrow focus on a single thing, such as the tai chi form, which combines movement and breath.

A trance state can be produced in various ways, such as by observing some type of repetitive rhythmic cue—watching a swinging pendulum, repeating a certain phrase over and over, or counting in a rhythmic fashion. You can observe this process in drumming circles when musicians gather, when kids dance in a mosh pit, or when someone is playing a sport such as tennis.

When most of us first learn to play tennis, our minds are clogged with rote details: watch the ball, turn your body, bring your racket back, hit the ball properly. Yet when you ask tennis pros what they were thinking just as they hit a great shot, they will usually tell you that they weren't thinking about anything—they had fallen into a trancelike state, dissociated from the environment, unaware of the crowd, oblivious to the last point or the next. They were in the moment.

Similarly, some forms of meditation induce a hypnotic state

to ward off distractions. This meditative state creates a number of health benefits, from lowering blood pressure to reducing anxiety.

RHYTHM AND MOVEMENT

When you combine movement with rhythm, you enjoy the double benefit of exercise and of a meditative state—and you lower CRP levels as well.

The simple combination of movement and rhythm creates new opportunities for dance that travel far beyond grabbing a partner for a basic waltz or a cha-cha. You can dance just by walking along a path. You can dance on a tennis court. You can dance by hiking, rowing, or biking. Any regular activity that combines rhythm and movement will help reduce immune activation and, in the process, the speed of aging.

Say you've come down with terrible back pain from a herniated disk. You're miserable and want relief. You're looking to pop a pill or get a numbing injection. Back pain is, in fact, the single most common reason why people are unable to go to work.

We used to think that when people strained or injured their back, the best thing to do was to put them on bed rest—no activity, no movement. Yet this prescription didn't seem to work; the pain didn't go away, and patients found themselves taking more and more pain medication without relief. Ultimately, they ended up in surgery. Too often that first surgery didn't work, and another operation was necessary. If that failed, a slippery slope loomed, and eventually a spinal fusion followed. (A spinal fusion is a process in which the cushion, or disk, between two vertebrae is removed and the bones of the spine are fused together using bone chips, completely immobilizing that section of the back.)

Medical scientists now know that advocating rest was bad advice. The dance of walking is preferred.

At first, such activity may be difficult because you feel so much pain, allowing limited mobility. But as you continue to walk, your body loosens up. Your immune activation level drops, and soon the pain improves.

When it comes to forms of dance, anything you can think of that combines movement with rhythm will be good. To get you started, following are some suggestions for dance exercises. Not only are they fun to do, but the more you do them, the longer and healthier your life.

TAKE ACTION: DANCE

FOR BEGINNERS

1. **Walking:** If you're just beginning a fitness program, start with the dance of walking. Try to get into a rhythm by walking at a steady pace for a fixed distance. Time yourself and keep a journal to monitor your progress.

   Depending on what kind of shape you're in when you start, choose a distance goal that you know you can achieve. Plan out a route around your neighborhood, or a number of laps around a track or at your local shopping mall (and that means walking, not shopping).

   The average person's objective should be to reach ten thousand steps (or about four miles) over the course of every day. It's very helpful to carry a pedometer, allowing you an easy way to keep track of your progress. Personally, I like the slim and unobtrusive Omron HJ-112 pedometer, which works whether you keep it in your pocket or purse, clipped on your belt, or around your neck. It also contains a memory function so you can check your daily steps for the past seven days. This simple tool helps motivate me to get in adequate walking every day.

   Remember that you're also trying to add some rhythm to

your steps. Don't walk unconsciously. Your legs, your arms—your entire body—should be involved in keeping the rhythm. Your walking should *feel* like a dance—and when you're in a rhythm, you'll likely find yourself singing or humming, or at least keeping time to a verse or beat in your head.

Think about all the rhythms that drill sergeants teach their recruits to help them march in sync. You too can create a marching song that keeps your tempo while you're walking, even if you sing it only in your head.

It's also important to fall into a regular walking schedule—and the sooner you make a regular habit of exercise, the more likely you are to keep exercising. Perhaps you can do it in the early morning, when the birds are chirping and few people are around. This will set a great tone for the day.

Also remember to wear comfortable walking shoes, such as sneakers or other supportive footwear. Avoid dress shoes, high heels, or work boots. If you suffer from foot problems such as fallen arches, weak ankles, or bunions, consult an expert about orthotics. Orthotics are inserts that slip into your walking shoes to correct foot or ankle-related problems. Everyone's feet are a bit different, and not every walking shoe on the shelf fits every foot. Podiatrists—and some shoe stores—use machines to analyze the pressure on your feet as you stand and walk, which allows them to prescribe a personalized orthotic shoe for you, just as an optometrist can prescribe glasses cut just so to correct your vision. Check with a podiatrist or sports medicine clinic, or search the yellow pages or the Internet for a computerized orthotics provider near you.

Of course, many people choose to do their walking on a treadmill in their home, office, or gym instead of outdoors, and that's fine. The treadmill belt is cushioned, so the impact isn't as harsh on your feet and legs as walking on a cement sidewalk or road.

2. **Low-impact options:** Walking isn't always your best dance option. If you have arthritis, bad knees, or are unable to walk for any other reason, find a different form of dance. The good news is that there are many other options for beginners.

    Swimming is an excellent choice—not only is it a great form of exercise, it's inherently rhythmic. Plus, there's no impact, nor any weight bearing, so swimming is a good option for those with joint problems. Even if you can't swim, you can try aerobic water dance. Most health clubs with a pool offer these classes, and they're usually led by trainers using upbeat music.

    Try to create a routine that you can regularly follow, such as a specific length of time and/or number of laps. Or spend a set amount of time doing water aerobics. Keep a record of your workouts to monitor your progress.

    Over time, you'll notice that you're able to do more with less effort. As you progress, you should either increase the length of your workouts or their intensity, so that you swim more laps in less time, or work out longer.

    If you don't have access to a pool, consider a low-impact exercise form, such as using an elliptical trainer. The machines provide a rhythmic nonimpact workout that doesn't strain knees, feet, or ankles. Some machines involve the arms and upper body, while others provide just a cardiovascular and lower-body workout.

3. **Entry-level aerobics:** Aerobics is another good beginners' exercise. Many classes are broadcast on TV, while others are available at your local health club or can be watched on VCR or DVD at home. The nice thing about doing aerobics at home is that you can take it at your own pace (although when you're in a class, the presence of the group can be highly motivating).

    Again, try to fall into a rhythm and routine. Set a specific time and duration for your sessions so you can create a lasting habit. Advance the duration and intensity of your workouts as you progress and improve.

4. **Basic ballroom dancing:** Don't forget to enjoy some actual dancing. Ballroom dancing satisfies the objectives of dance—movement to rhythm. Not only that, it requires coordination and unspoken communication with your partner. And because your mind has to be focused on what you're doing—or you may stumble or fall behind—it's also a form of moving meditation. Try it. You'll like it!

FOR INTERMEDIATES

1. **Biking:** Naturally rhythmic, with an obvious cadence, biking is an excellent way to add dance to your UltraLongevity program. Road, mountain, tandem, and even stationary upright and recumbent bikes are all effective.

   If you're outdoors, find a bicycle path, since riding alongside cars can be dangerous. Always wear a helmet as well as other protective gear, including bicycling gloves and padded shorts. If you can't find a safe place and good gear, consider an indoor stationary bike.

2. **Rowing:** This is one of the most rhythmic forms of exercise, and one of the healthiest—as noted, tests show that rowers enjoy some of the lowest CRP levels of all athletes. Like biking, rowing is flexible. It can be done outdoors in a real boat, or indoors on a rowing machine; either is fine. Start with an experienced trainer who can show you the proper form and technique so you begin with good habits. Use music, or even a metronome, to keep your rhythm.

3. Jogging: For those of us with good knees, jogging is a great form of rhythmic exercise. It presents opportunities for new places, fresh views, and for putting your mind in a state of peaceful focus. It can be done practically anywhere and doesn't require much in the way of specialized equipment. You can easily track your progress if you use some type of speed and distance device. My favorite is the Nike + iPod Sport Kit, which allows Nike+ shoes and an iPod nano to work together as a combination pedometer, speed and distance monitor, and music player.

4. Jumping rope: Here is another great form of rhythmic aerobic movement. Trainers have long recognized rope jumping's potential, which is why it is used to cross-train all types of athletes, from boxers to gymnasts. It's fun, requires concentration, and is naturally rhythmic. It may even remind you of your glory days on the school playground, chanting dozens of jump rope songs while showing off with your friends.

Jumping rope can be done just about anywhere, and it doesn't require fancy equipment. If you need help getting started, ask your kids, relatives, or friends. It's amazing how well jumping rope has stood up over time despite all the technology that surrounds us—all you need is a rope, some music, and some energy.

5. Tap, hip-hop, and square dancing: These are all aerobic forms of dance that bubble with rhythm, can improve your fitness, and will put a smile on your face. Take a class, get a tape, or join a group, but just do it!

When the subject of tap dancing comes up, patients often respond, "I've always wanted to learn to do that." What are you waiting for? Now's the time. Plus, if you register for a class that's held, say, twice a week, you're much more apt to keep the appointment, which will help you to hold to a steady routine.

FOR MORE ADVANCED DANCERS

1. **Competitive sports:** Sports such as tennis, racquetball, volleyball, competitive running, or gymnastics all require a high level of physical fitness and coordination. They are not for people just starting an exercise program, but if you're fit enough, they can boost your dance program to the next level due to the strength, endurance, agility, and balance required. Combined with rhythm, these attributes provide health rewards in addition to personal satisfaction and enjoyment. Find a coach or partner who can guide your progress to reach your goals.

2. **Martial arts:** The martial arts arise from a centuries-old tradition combining movement and rhythm, and include karate, tae kwon do, jujitsu, and simple tai chi, among other forms. Martial arts stress the mind-body connection and require concentration and mindfulness in movement.

    I can recall my own son, Tim, learning Okinawa karate. The concentration, balance, mindfulness, and rhythmic motion instilled into him as a young child have carried over into his other activities as a teen. Like Tim, once you learn these basics, you can apply them to almost all sports involving movement and rhythm.

    Practicing martial arts doesn't necessarily mean fighting, or even defending yourself. Tai chi is a mindful moving meditation derived from ancient martial arts practices of China, and yet its purpose is promoting inner peace and health. Eastern cultures have long recognized the connection between a strong body and a strong, calm mind.

3. **Hiking:** Although hiking can be strenuous, especially in rugged terrain, there are few rhythmic activities as rewarding. The serenity of pristine environments and the sense of accomplish-

ment in reaching remote and scenic vistas can be among life's greatest pleasures. It's usually not feasible to go hiking on a daily basis, but occasional hiking trips are well worth pursuing.

Staying in shape for strenuous hiking requires a regular training program. Don't forget to wear sturdy shoes. I also recommend hiking poles to prevent falls and injuries and to foster upper-body conditioning as you hike.

4. **Interval training:** One of the most strenuous and yet physically rewarding forms of exercise, interval training involves periods of very strenuous exercise alternating with periods of moderate exercise. By pushing the workout intensity to near-maximal levels for short bursts, interspersed with your usual, moderate exercise regime, you can dramatically improve your overall fitness level and health.

   This kind of training can be done during almost any kind of exercise, whether it's jogging, swimming, biking, or rowing. It simply requires that you add spurts of anaerobic exercise during your regular aerobic workout. "Anaerobic" means that your muscles require more oxygen than your heart and lungs can deliver. During anaerobic exercise, your muscles build up lactic acid and develop what's known as oxygen debt, which has to be repaid with a period of rest and increased breathing.

   Interval training is only for the physically fit. If you have any concerns or questions, check with your physician, and work with a personal trainer who can give you individualized guidelines.

5. **Strenuous dance forms:** Jitterbug, African dance, polkas, ballet, and other forms of highly strenuous dance are among the most entertaining of all dances, but also require the greatest effort. Most communities have classes in at least some of these athletic forms of dance, and making such a commitment is a

great way to keep yourself and your dance program on track. Even if you're in great shape, don't be surprised if an hour of jitterbugging leaves you sweaty and exhausted. It will also leave you feeling terrific.

The list of dance exercises outlined here is by no means comprehensive, but it should clue you in to the wide range of possibilities, as well as what to keep in mind when you attempt to slow the aging process and deactivate your immune system by combining rhythm and movement.

If you wish, you can invent an exercise program that's just right for you. For example, one of my patients and his friends throw the Frisbee around in his backyard to a pulsating beat from a CD player, creating a self-invented ballet of hip-hop catch. Another patient turns up her stereo, jumps into her lap pool, and walks to the beat in the water—a much more strenuous form of walking than on land. Still another patient loves doing jumping jacks to 1970s disco music in his apartment. It makes him happy, it makes his heart happy, and it makes his immune system happy. Who could ask for more?

STEP 5: LOVE

WHENEVER I DISCUSS breathing, eating, and sleeping, everyone is quickly on board. But talking about love can cause some people to feel uncomfortable. They look as if they want to say, as the Tina Turner song lyric goes, "What's love got to do with it?"

The answer is, when you're talking about health, love has a lot to do with it. So if for some reason the topic of love makes you uneasy, reflect a moment. Is love an uncomfortable or painful theme for you to consider? Have you lost a loved one, or the feeling of being loved? Do you discount the power of love? Are you harboring feelings of anger, worry, or despair, or do you lack self-esteem?

If you feel this way, so does your immune system, and the pain could be eating away at your health. Your immune system feels whatever you feel. So if you are experiencing soothing and nurturing emotions, it knows this and responds in kind.

By the word "love," I don't necessarily mean a warm one-on-one relationship with another person. Love is a vast and open-ended sensation, the most written-about, talked-about, and worried-about emotion in the history of humankind, and can be expressed in countless ways.

Love can mean love of nature. It can mean a feeling of oneness with the world. It can denote that warm, fuzzy emotion you have when doing something as simple as appreciating a cozy fireplace on a cold morning, or the more complicated sensations that accompany a brand-new relationship.

Love is beautiful and universal. Love is a deep sense of appreciation, understanding, sympathy, and empathy. Love is the appreciation of connectedness, whether that connection is to a partner, a child, a parent, a friend, a community, or Mother Earth.

Love is the antidote to hate, anger, fear, and sadness. It's hard to feel these negative emotions when you feel love. But when people sense negative emotions, their bodies sense them too. The immune system is particularly attuned to our emotional state, which means both negative and positive emotions play a role in our health patterns.

Scientific research is continually confirming the links between negative emotions and disease conditions and accelerated aging. For example, hostility has been linked with heart disease—even in the young. The results of the CARDIA Study (Coronary Artery Risk Development in Young Adults) of 374 people between eighteen and thirty years old showed that higher levels of hostility increased the risk of a significant amount of calcified plaque accumulating in the coronary arteries by almost tenfold (JAMA, May 17, 2000). In this same study, nonloving feelings such as hostility were also shown to predict the development of high blood pressure years later (JAMA, October 22, 2003).

Happy, loving people tend to be healthier. Of course, there have been several challenges to this kind of research, because it's entirely possible that people may be happier *because* they are healthier. But in a review of research performed over the past ten years, Professor Sheldon Cohen and postdoctoral student Sarah Pressman of Carnegie Mellon University concluded that emotions such as love are indeed strongly linked to both good health and longevity (*Psychological Bulletin*, December 12, 2004).

Likewise, in a 2005 presentation to the Brisbane, Australia, health and aging conference, Marc Cohen, professor of complementary medicine at the Royal Melbourne Institute of Technology, noted, "There's a growing research base that suggests the more we experience love in our life the longer we will live and the more protected we are against a whole lot of degenerative diseases."

ACCEPTANCE

One of the most important aspects of emotional health is acceptance—being able to trust the world and to accept your place within it.

This is not easy to do. There are so many things that can upset us, from current events to problems among our friends and family. Yet being able to function on a day-to-day basis without letting bad news, world events, or politics make you miserable is important to your health.

While some people might react to a difficult situation with anger or anxiety, another person might respond completely differently, accepting it as just another one of life's challenges.

It's particularly important to learn acceptance when dealing with your health. During my training in oncology, I worked with a professor who had an uncanny ability to predict which patients would breeze through their cancer treatments and which wouldn't.

When I asked him how he knew, he replied that he studied attitude. Patients prone to agonize over every detail of therapy, and to analyze every possible cause of each of their symptoms, would magnify the side effects from their treatment. Patients who more easily accepted their diagnosis seemed to sail through without a hitch. This didn't necessarily translate into better long-term outcomes, but it did predict how patients tolerated their therapy at the time.

Still another part of the puzzle of acceptance and love might best be defined as inner peace. This attitude can arise from faith, from a spiritual belief system, or from a high degree of self-knowledge. Its sources are few, but its rewards are bountiful.

People who possess this kind of peace find they are better able to deal with stress than those who don't. Studies have shown, for example, that a personal belief system helps reduce side effects from radiation therapy for cancer (*Strahlentherapie und Onkologie*, May 2006). And in a study of the autoimmune disease rheumatoid arthritis, patients who felt love in the form of someone praying for them showed significant overall improvement in arthritis during a one-year follow-up. This beneficial effect was found only if the person who was praying was actually present with the patient during prayer. Praying from a distance (known as intercessory prayer) didn't seem to provide a benefit. Figuratively speaking, the immune system had to feel the love in person (*Southern Medical Journal*, December 2000).

LOVE OF NATURE

Perhaps one of the most extraordinary kinds of love is an appreciation for the wonder of nature and for the awesome interconnections between all the facets of the world.

Just today we had a stunningly lovely summer afternoon here in the Berkshires of western Massachusetts. The heat and humidity had built up during the day and then broke during a wonderful, soothing hour-long rain. My daughter, Brenna, and I sat on the front porch, and both of us watched, awestruck, the phenomenon of rain. Little droplets of water, falling out of the sky, bringing cool, clean liquid that nourishes all of the grass, plants, and trees, collecting in small streams and rivulets, carrying away dust and debris, cleansing and rinsing, then ultimately flowing into rivers and the ocean, where it nourishes and renews the algae, insects, and fish in a complex cycle that is so perfect it's miraculous, and yet also so simple. Water falling from heaven.

Sometimes it seems as though the diversity of life is like the most intricate of musical fugues. Just as Johann Sebastian Bach took a single motif and changed it a hundred different ways to produce a startling orchestral creation, so too with life itself. We see a motif and then a multitude of variations on it. We notice a single sparrow but then consider that there are dozens of varieties of sparrow, each with a slightly different beak, wing, call, eye, and niche in which to live.

That same pattern is repeated countless times for all the diversity of life on the planet. It's incredible and complex, awesome and beautiful, this world of ours. How can you not feel love for nature? And when you do, you're telling the immune system that everything is copasetic—stay cool, calm, and healthy.

INTERPERSONAL LOVE

If this kind of appreciation of nature isn't your favorite source of love, perhaps another person is.

Do you remember the old Charlton Heston movie *The Omega Man?* The action took place after the world's population had been killed during intense biological warfare. As the recipient of an experimental vaccine, Heston's character seems to be the last survivor of humankind, which is why he is the Omega man.

For a while he enjoys his time alone, driving different cars, watching movies, eating whatever foods he desires. But what he discovers—when he's not fighting off the undead and other postapocalyptic horrors—is that he really wants another person with whom to share his existence. What good is a long life spent all alone?

There are countless ways to feel love when you're with someone else. You may see him or her smiling at you. You might remember a multitude of different ways that person shows you love, whether it's through a kiss, a touch, or just a parting glance.

Interpersonal love heals. Lovers live longer. A study by the Centers for Disease Control from December 2004 polled more than 120,000 adults and found that married people are more likely to be in good health than unmarried ones, and are less likely to smoke, drink, or be sedentary. This doesn't apply to every marriage (and certainly being married does not always imply the presence of love), but there is a clear trend for better health, longevity, and self-care behavior patterns among those with a partner.

A study of 490 women by Linda Gallo, PhD, as reported in the September 2003 issue of *Health Psychology*, showed that women who were in satisfying relationships (whether married or not) had lower blood pressure, lower cholesterol levels, and lower body mass index than women who weren't.

On the other hand, people who have experienced pain in relationships suffer more than just emotional pain. Medical science has proven the existence of a broken heart; the term is "stress cardiomyopathy." In a study reported in the *New England Journal of Medicine* in February 2005, severe heart dysfunction was observed in nineteen patients who had felt sudden emotional stress, or a broken heart. Symptoms included chest pain, electrocardiogram (EKG) signs similar to those of a heart attack, shortness of breath, and even heart failure.

What's interesting is that biopsies showed that the patient's immune system was actually attacking the heart—macrophages (MPs) had infiltrated the heart muscle, causing wanton destruction and damage. This damage was found to be reversible, however; with time, the immune system retreated and the heart function returned to normal.

Being in a high-quality relationship has also been found to be protective for the heart. In a study of 393 women participating in the Healthy Women Study, a high-quality relationship seemed to protect women from coronary artery disease (*Psychosomatic Medicine*, November/December 2003).

DON'T FORGET TO LOVE YOURSELF

Here's another thought about love: You need to love yourself. Yet love for oneself is often the hardest form to find. Many people feel they don't deserve to be loved—by others or by themselves.

Let's nip that idea right in the bud. Although it might be easy to get down on yourself, remember that we are all struggling with exactly the same challenges and foibles. Being human means being imperfect. We also share many emotions and desires in common: we want to be happy, we want to be loved, and we want to love others. Once we realize we are all in the same boat, it becomes easier to feel compassion toward others and toward ourselves.

If people realized that self-regard might improve their health, it might prompt them to try harder to be their own best and most loving friend.

Social connectedness improves health and longevity, and social isolation increases mortality. A study of 2,575 adults older than age sixty-five, as reported in the journal *Epidemiology* (September 1997), revealed that those with few social contacts over a three-year period experienced higher mortality than people with richer, more frequent social connections. People who increased the number of social contacts from few to many experienced an improvement in survival and reduction in mortality comparable to that of highly sociable people.

One of my own patients, Marcia, is a perfect example of the effect of love on health. Marcia battles with her weight, blood pressure, cholesterol, and self-esteem. All of these indicators track together, precisely and predictably in concert with Marcia's love life.

Unmarried, in her late forties, Marcia is the primary caretaker for her aging parents. She has essentially sacrificed her life to that single duty; her work, her own home, and her relationships have all taken secondary positions. As a result, Marcia has struggled to maintain long-term, loving relationships.

Over the years, Marcia has had several relationships, but they don't last. Still, in the first few weeks of romance, as she falls in love, the physical signs are impressive. Marcia immediately loses weight—the pounds seem to melt off. When she enters my office, her mood is lighter; she's smiling and joking. Her blood pressure is lower than usual and her blood work also shows improvement— lower cholesterol, lower triglycerides, and lower CRP. Marcia's immune system loves it when she's in love.

But when the relationship ends, Marcia's health problems return.

HOW MUCH LOVE CAN FIT IN A DAY?

Some people might go an afternoon, or a week, or a month without experiencing love. But the experience of love should be a daily event.

Many people wake up in the morning, grab their cup of coffee, answer dozens of e-mails, read the paper, rush off to work, get into a traffic jam, dash up to the office, deal with all the problems on their desk, wolf down a business lunch, get stuck in meetings, rush home, eat a fast dinner, answer more e-mails, watch the news, and finally fall into bed.

What happened to love? People remember to brush their teeth; why can't they remember to experience a little love?

I don't think anybody hasn't had at least a brief experience of love in his or her life. We don't need to teach people to know love as much as we have to remind them to feel it—because almost none of us get enough.

Despite all we know about love, and how good it is for us, our society doesn't accord love the value it deserves. I'm convinced people would benefit greatly from thinking about value in terms other than simply money. Wouldn't it be wonderful if instead of thinking about someone's financial net worth, we thought about, say, someone's net compassion?

In the small Asian country Bhutan, the government doesn't spend a great amount of time worrying about its gross national product. Instead, they talk about what they call gross national happiness. That's their currency—happiness. It means more to them than money.

This is one reason Bhutan permits only a limited number of tourists into the country. They don't want their people to be influenced by the Western way of thinking.

Interestingly, but not surprisingly, the chief causes of death in Bhutan include none of the diseases we see so often in the United States, such as cancer, heart disease, and Alzheimer's. Instead, they are bacterial and viral diseases such as respiratory tract infections, skin and parasitic infections, and malaria. Like the United States a hundred years ago, Bhutan has yet to benefit from the advances against infectious diseases. Imagine how combining modern advances in treating infections with Bhutan's attitude of happiness might affect human longevity and aging there. Remember Shangri-la, the mythical land from *Lost Horizon*, where the citizens lived healthy lives forever? It was set near Bhutan, in the Himalayas; perhaps the author knew something we don't.

In my own practice, love is one of my most common "prescriptions"; we call it Vitamin L. Often my patients have so much—money, freedom, good jobs, fancy homes—but they lack the most important asset: love. Because of this, they often feel anxious, sad, or even angry.

My prescription to you is Vitamin L. It's easy to say, and of course, finding the kind of love you most desire is not simple. That's why we provide easy-to-follow exercises that can help patients (and you) find love in your life—almost anywhere and at any time. Remember, you don't need a romantic relationship—hidden possibilities for love exist everywhere. Perhaps you enjoy a walk around the reservoir on a spring morning, a bike ride out in the country, or a cup of coffee with a good friend. One of my patients in Manhattan spends a few minutes each day outside the local doggy day care center, watching the puppies play. How can you feel pressured and rushed if you've just watched a dozen dogs having the time of their lives?

The point of this chapter isn't to make you a loving person in ten minutes. It takes a lifetime of work to be loving. But we can always improve our loving skills. We can discover the love within us that we've kept hidden; at worst, we can move from being a person who feels no love at all to someone who can feel at least a little.

TAKE ACTION: LOVE

Do you really have to learn what love is? I doubt it. Each of us arrives on earth with love as built-in, standard equipment, but for countless reasons we sometimes forget about love, or choose to forget, or fall out of practice.

As I say, like breathing, love is often overlooked, denied, or underappreciated as a powerful agent for health and healing. Perhaps you've given up on love, or were hurt by it, or have it in your life but don't communicate, strengthen, or spread it.

But even if love has atrophied, it can be revived and renewed, as long as you want to restore it. The following exercises and techniques can help remind you how to love, and can strengthen the love you already possess. With practice and conscious attention, you will improve and feel a stronger sense of love that's easier to engage. After all, to get really good at something requires training.

The important thing is to do something. Don't read this chapter and procrastinate. Take steps now.

1. **Consider therapy:** If you're feeling bereft of love, one route to recapture it is to enter psychotherapy. Personally, I recommend cognitive behavioral therapy, a model that I value for working on specific psychological and interpersonal issues. It can truly help people begin to experience love.

   "Cognitive" refers to thought—this type of therapy helps people change the way they think. For example, many of us have recurring negative thoughts that block our ability to experience love. We may think, "I'm a bad person," "The world is terrible," or "I always get the blame." Such thoughts are inaccurate generalizations that obstruct the ability to experience love.

   The cognitive behavioral therapy model helps people analyze and deconstruct these unsupportive thoughts and then change the way they think about their lives. By shifting from a negative thought pattern to a more accurate and positive one, people allow love into their thoughts.

   This is the beginning of the process. With practice, almost anyone can learn to change his or her thinking to allow for, and encourage, love and compassion.

   Many other excellent therapeutic solutions exist, from standard Freudian psychiatry to primal scream therapy. Whichever you choose, now is the time to start.

2. **Speak up:** Tell someone you love him or her. We often forget during our day-to-day routine that people can't read our minds. If you don't express how you feel, no one may ever know. We all need to communicate, to let people know what's going on inside our hearts.

   Also, when you tell someone "I love you," you'll almost

always receive an expression of love in return. An interchange of "I love you" with "I love you too" can be better for your health than any supplement or medication.

3. **Get a pet:** Abundant research has demonstrated the superb health benefits of pet ownership. Pet owners generally enjoy better moods, lower blood pressure, less incidence of heart disease, lower cholesterol, and improved immune system function, to name just a few benefits. Pet ownership, especially during childhood, also seems to reduce the risk of allergies and asthma.

4. **Keep a love journal:** Moments of love often pass by in our lives without comment and, sometimes, without notice. Many people keep journals, but too often we scribble in them only when things are going badly. One of my patients says that nearly every entry in his long series of journals starts off with, "Just when I thought things couldn't get worse . . ."

It doesn't matter where or how you do it, whether you prefer to write longhand in a beautifully bound blank book or type on a computer screen, it's helpful to keep a daily diary of every "love incident" that passes your way. This could mean anything from a spouse's kind words to a cat's purr, from a stranger's random compliment to a purposeful accolade at work—or even just a private moment when you glanced at a garden and took in its extraordinary beauty.

Making a note of these moments can help sustain you when you're feeling bereft. After you write them down, you may discover that more of them occur than you expected.

5. **Remind-a-love:** You tape a note on the back door reminding yourself to pick up an item at the grocery store. You stick a Post-it on the refrigerator so you won't forget a doctor's appointment.

Think about doing something similar with love. Give yourself a daily love reminder. When I turn on my computer in the morning, I don't want the news. Current events are important, but wouldn't it be great if somebody sent me a message of love first?

Set up your computer to run a continuous slide show of favorite photographs that remind you of loving times. Send your loved ones a daily e-mail reminding them of how much you care; encourage a response to keep the love flowing. Enter pop-up reminders in your calendar to tell yourself that you are loved and to share the love with someone else. Make these reminders daily, weekly, or monthly.

6. **Read a book:** A book can be almost anything you want it to be: a stirring adventure, a gripping mystery, or a thought-provoking journey. In the context of love, books on the subject can be a terrific way to learn how to cultivate it.

Personally, I am fond of books with loving, inspirational messages, particularly those that contain concise passages with easily extractable messages. Maybe there's a paragraph, or a sentence, or even just a few words that you can use as a mantra, an inspirational passage that helps prompt your mindset toward a more positive outlook for the rest of the day.

The book currently lying next to my bed is *The Art of Happiness: A Handbook for Living,* by the Dalai Lama, and it's replete with inspirational affirmations. Other wonderful books that can help you understand love include *Man's Search for Meaning,* by Viktor Frankl; *On Caring,* by Milton Mayeroff; *Peace Is Every Step,* by Thich Nhat Hanh; *The Prophet,* by Kahlil Gibran; *What Happy People Know,* by Dan Baker; and *Love Is the Killer App,* by Tim Sanders.

The books don't have to be nonfiction. Sometimes a novel can be a wonderful introduction to love. Think of some of the great novels of all time, such as *Anna Karenina*, or recent best-sellers like *Cold Mountain*.

One of the best parts of reading is that you can do it whenever you want, wherever you want, and you can read it over and over again. Now that's love!

7. **Watch a movie:** Movies, too, can provide insight into compassion. For example, *Groundhog Day*, a 1993 comedy, is taught in colleges and seminars around the country as a lesson in empathy. The main character, a vain weatherman, has to relive the same day over and over until he can finally feel something for someone other than himself.

One of my favorite movies of all time is *Hook*, the Hollywood sequel to *Peter Pan*. In it, Peter Pan returns to his childhood roots after growing up and forgetting how to fly. He relearns flying by remembering the secret—all he had to do was think about something he loved. He thought about his children, and the next moment he was zipping through the air with the greatest of ease.

Other movies that teach lessons about love include *Moonstruck*, *The Joy Luck Club*, *Driving Miss Daisy*, *Good Will Hunting*, and *Brokeback Mountain*, along with hundreds more. As long as there is love, Hollywood will never stop making films about it.

8. **Use a love mantra:** A love mantra is a word or phrase you repeat to yourself to remind you of connectedness and compassion. I have one patient who was so moved by the story of Bhutan that her mantra is "Compassion is the currency."

Whenever someone says or does something to anger you, instead of feeling anger, repeat your love mantra. Some people might use the biblical "Turn the other cheek"; others chant

"We all are one." Another favorite is the title of the old Beatles song "All You Need Is Love."

9. **Take a love breath:** In the Breathe step, I discussed exhalation and the exhalation plateau. What I call the love breath takes place when you take in a long, deep breath; as you're inhaling, repeat to yourself, "I love breathing in." On exhalation say, "I love breathing out." With repetition, this short exercise transforms into a mantra of "I love all the time" and "I love living."

As mentioned, people forget what a pleasure breathing truly is. Imagine if you were always fighting for breath, as people with breathing disorders have to do. Breathing is life's simplest but most profound joy, yet it is taken for granted. Breathe. Appreciate. Live. Love.

10. **Smell the roses:** Life's little details deserve appreciation. The wonder of it all lies in the details, and then the details within the details: flowers with delicate, specialized parts designed to attract insects and encourage pollination, leaves with tiny pores that allow the plants to breathe in carbon dioxide and breathe out oxygen. The cooling breeze that feels so good on your face is a miracle in itself—how would it feel if the air were always still? Don't forget the beauty of dusk as the sun sets, or dawn as it rises. Everyday occurrences present endless opportunities to feel love. Make a list of details you take for granted, and you'll come up with hundreds more.

11. **Be creative:** Find interesting ways to spread your love. For instance, I know a doctor in Manhattan who leaves money on subway platforms. It makes going down into the subway more interesting for him and means that someone that day is going to be surprised.

Along the same lines, my wife, Siobhan, and I used to have a favorite hiking trail in the White Mountains of New Hampshire. We loved it for the huge rocks we'd pass; when you looked in the rocks, you'd find countless little burrows filled with moss and plants. We always joked that they looked like tiny leprechaun homes. So one day we brought a few miniature porcelain leprechauns and set them up inside some of the burrows, so that someday someone might look and be surprised.

12. **Join a support group:** Bountiful research on support groups shows how they can positively impact the course of cancer therapy and of treatment for autoimmune diseases such as AIDS. People in support groups display fewer side effects and complications, and tolerate their treatment better, than those who aren't in these groups.

You don't have to have a health condition to provide support. All you have to do is be open and available to support others. Indeed, support groups aren't only for the ill or the bereaved. There are support groups for just about everything, whether it's SAD (seasonal affective disorder) or compulsive shopping. Whatever is holding you back, you can meet people who feel similarly. Together you will be stronger than you are alone.

13. **Become an advocate:** If you have strong feelings about an issue, whether it's animals, the environment, or politics, share those feelings with the world. We all know about commitment in the context of a relationship, but sometimes committing yourself to your love of something other than another person can bring out the best in you.

There is certainly no shortage of important issues for which each of us could become an advocate. It's also possible that in working for a cause, you might find a soul mate with whom you can share love.

Similarly, volunteering to help others is one of the most powerful expressions of love. If compassion is the new wealth, then the opportunity to help someone is the new currency. What goes around comes around. Those invested in helping others will find friends at their side in times of need.

STEP 6: SOOTHE

AS YOU NOW well know, the immune system has evolved to defend and protect us from a dangerous world. If we lived in a bubble, or if life took place in a germ-free utopia, there would be no need for an immune system. However, it's a jungle out there, with entire ecosystems of creatures whose existence depends on their ability to harm us. Our daily environment is dangerous, and the more threatening it becomes, the more reactive our immune system.

This chapter is about how you can help your immune system by creating an external world as soothing and healthy as possible. If your environment is calm and nurturing, the immune system won't become overly defensive.

The womb is a good example of such a place. Inside the protective, peaceful environment of a healthy womb, there are no perceived threats. An ample cushion of amniotic fluid protects and surrounds the developing fetus. Shocks, bumps, and pressure are buffered or eliminated. Temperature is constant. The placenta supplies a steady stream of nurturing oxygen and nutrients. Relaxing hormones such as progesterone and oxytocin bathe the mother's own brain and immune system, creating a feeling of love and peace within her body.

As a result, a newborn baby's immune system is underdeveloped; as mentioned earlier, it takes at least three months after birth for it to function well on its own, without help from the passive immunity provided by the mother's antibodies.

However, if complications occur during a pregnancy, the situation changes. Injury, premature labor, bleeding, or placental problems all can transform the uterus's normally peaceful environment. Research shows that complicated pregnancies create a much higher risk not only for the mother, but also for the baby, who is typically born smaller than normal, with an overactive immune system. In fact, one predictor of an overactive immune system as an adult is having suffered through a stressed gestation.

Researchers at Glasgow University's MIDSPAN Family Study showed that CRP levels in adults are inversely related to birth weight. In other words, the smaller you were at birth, the higher your CRP level later in life.

In fact, adult CRP levels are increased about 10 percent for every 2 pounds less than 9½ pounds a baby weighs. Seven-and-a-half pound babies had CRP levels 10 percent higher and 5½-pound babies had CRP levels 20 percent higher than 9½-pounders.

You may have heard stories of children who must live in protective bubbles. Rare disorders such as SCID (severe combined immunodeficiency disease) block these children's ability to develop a functional immune system; they are utterly vulnerable to any of the myriad germs in the environment. Their only chance for survival is to avoid all contact with the outside world until a lifesaving bone marrow transplant can be performed.

Luckily, most of us don't have to live in a bubble, but we can all profit from exerting control over our external environment, which should be as stress free, calming, and free of infectious threats and harmful toxins as possible. By so doing, we can soothe our immune system, reduce immune activation, and slow aging.

HOME

For starters, you spend most of your time at home, so make it a safe and peaceful place. You should always feel "at home" when you're at home.

When I think about a happy, soothing home environment, I picture Bilbo Baggins's house in *The Lord of the Rings*. His house perfectly fit its hobbit inhabitant—the round doors, the low ceilings, the warm hearth, the root vegetables hanging from the ceiling, the thick wooden table, the hobbit-sized stools, the worn but nice-looking wood floor. Bilbo's home had an excellent hobbit feng shui. It was so welcoming, warm, and safe-feeling, I know I could live in such a home—at least, if I were a hobbit.

That's the way your own home should feel to you.

Your house doesn't have to be big, lavish, or fancy; it just needs to feel homey. You've probably heard of the TV show *Extreme Makeover: Home Edition,* in which builders perform a complete home renovation. The special touches they create to make each home personal and meaningful to its owners are the best part of the makeover.

Make your home peaceful, with pictures on the wall that are calming to view, colors that are relaxing, chairs that feel comfortable.

Lighting is also important. Your home should let in natural light, allowing for a full spectrum that neither incandescent nor fluorescent lights can provide. (You can also buy full-spectrum light-bulbs, which provide a richer spectrum of light and can replace standard incandescent bulbs.) And just as it's important to make your bedroom as dark as possible at night, you should let in as much light as possible during the daytime, and keep windows open to let the fresh air flow through.

TOUCH

Touch is an often-overlooked part of wellness. Yet touch cements a bond between a mother and child, husband and wife, friend and friend. Even when we first meet, our instinct is to touch the other with a handshake. The immune system responds to touch because it conveys a message of peace, calm, and relaxation.

It's not just humans who rely on social touch for their well-being. Go to any zoo and you'll witness many species of animals touching each other. For example, chimpanzees frequently groom one another, picking off lice or nits, or just brushing and combing through hairs. This very social interaction is a crucial part of development and communication for the chimps' immune system. A monkey in a social group will have a much healthier immune system than a monkey who's been isolated.

Touch is one of the best means of encouraging the sense of community and relaxation that soothes the immune system. Countless ways exist to engage in touch, such as massage, which comes in many varieties. For example, at Canyon Ranch, we offer more than twenty different types, including Ayurvedic, craniosacral, deep tissue, Lomi Lomi Hawaiian, hot stone, Jin Shin Jyutsu, myofascial, neuromuscular, polarity, reflexology, shiatsu, Swedish, Watsu, and zero balancing.

Research shows that massage improves natural killer cell activity (a Miami School of Medicine study, revealing a significant increase in NK cell number and activity after daily massages for one month, was reported in the *International Journal of Neuroscience*, February 1996.) As mentioned earlier, natural killer cells are involved in killing cancer cells, cell DNA mutations, and cells infected with viruses or other immune system disorders, from HIV to lupus to rheumatoid arthritis. We want NK cells to flourish in our body. Massage can accomplish this goal.

Another form of therapeutic touch is known as healing touch. Healing-touch practitioners are often nurses who provide caring, compassion, and healing thoughts, which they channel in the form of gentle touch. Many healing-touch practitioners use the chakra system, a form of Eastern medicine involving energy channels, to help guide their touch therapy.

According to studies, patients undergoing healing-touch therapy experience improvements in pain, anxiety, depression, and overall well-being. Therapeutic touch is also used in nurseries to calm irritable newborns.

Still one more form of therapeutic touch can support the immune system: sexuality. Research has shown that sexual arousal increases the number of natural killer cells in the blood (*Neuro-ImmunoModulation*, 2004). A study of almost thirty thousand men (published in JAMA, April 2004) found that frequency of ejaculation was proportional to reduced risk of prostate cancer: men reporting more than twenty-one ejaculations per month were found to have a lower risk of this cancer. The reason for this association wasn't clear, but it's possible that frequent ejaculation may reduce the likelihood of chronic prostate infections that might cause prostate cancer.

Swedish scientists found that men who stopped having sexual intercourse died sooner than those who continued; a North Carolina research team also found that the men who had the most intercourse tended to live longer. Part of the reason for this may be explained by this study: Scientists at Pennsylvania's Wilkes University surveyed students' sex lives and assessed their levels of immunoglobulin A, another indicator of the immune system's strength. Students who reported one or two sexual encounters a week had 30 percent more of the protective antibody than those who were celibate.

SMELL

Another means of soothing the immune system is through the sense of smell.

Odors exert a powerful impact on the immune system. Anatomically speaking, the nose is the closest connection between the brain and the outside world; the cribriform plate, the bone between the nose and the brain, is the thinnest bone in the base of the skull, and the easiest to break.

Directly through the cribriform plate travels the olfactory nerve, which is responsible for sensing odors that proceed right from the nose to the brain; there's no quicker way of transmitting information to the brain than by smelling it.

Smell's importance probably derives from the evolutionary needs of our ancestors, whose sense of smell was critical for their survival—they had to be able to find food, and test it for safety, using their nose. Today, most animals have a much more highly developed sense of smell than humans. Professionally trained tracking dogs such as bloodhounds can capture someone's scent from sniffing just a few shed skin cells. Dogs are now being used in health care to sense oncoming epileptic attacks in patients by smelling a change in body chemistry; similarly, it now appears that dogs can sniff out cancer too.

Where our olfactory world is equivalent to low-resolution black-and-white TV, an animal's world of smell is like a Technicolor movie.

Research has demonstrated the ability of scents to induce relaxation and to lift mood. Aromatherapy, or the healing use of smells, is employed worldwide in treating a number of psychological conditions, including depression, stress, insomnia, anxiety, and drug and nicotine dependence.

Scientific research suggests that different aromas have different effects—some calming, some arousing—and that these effects are different in men and women. Lavender, a mild sedative for men, is a stimulant for women (*Chronobiology International*, 2005).

Even premature babies respond to pleasant aromas; premies in hospital incubators had 36 percent fewer apneas (breath-holding spells) than control infants when a pleasant aroma was added to the incubator (*Pediatrics*, January 2005).

Because smell has been such an important sense in human evolution, alerting us to dangers such as smoke, rotten food, or poison (and also to possible mates and other good things), your sense of smell is still a vital cue to tell your immune system to respond or relax.

SOUND

Yet another of our senses can soothe the immune system: hearing.

Sound can be used therapeutically in many ways—playing or listening to music, chanting, singing, sounding gongs—and research shows that these sounds have positive effects on the immune system. For example, in one study, mice with cancer that were exposed to five hours of music during the day had a better antitumor immune response than mice that did not hear music (*Life Sciences*, July 2002).

In human blood studies, listening to music has been shown to reduce the levels of immune-activating cytokines, including interleukin-6, while increasing endorphins, morphinelike natural chemicals made by the brain and immune system (*Medical Science Monitor*, June 10, 2004).

Interestingly, people who suffer from hearing loss have higher levels of immune activation than people with normal hearing. Not being able to hear well is stressful. Research published in *Aviation, Space, and Environmental Medicine* (March 1999) showed higher levels of circulating T cells in patients with damaged hearing due to loud noise exposure.

Music therapy is an effective, inexpensive, and pleasing way of modulating the immune response without causing any side effects. So let the music play!

CLEAN AIR

Keeping our external environment sanitary is another way to reduce immune activation.

People generally assume the air they breathe is clean unless smoke or smog is patently noticeable. Yet studies show that air pollution is actually much worse indoors than outdoors, although few of us ever perceive this. Worldwide, indoor air pollution ranks as one of the leading causes of death in children; in fact, in 2004 the primary cause was acute respiratory infections, to which air pollution was a major contributor. Indoor stoves fueled by dung, brush, and wood are used for cooking for more than half the world's population; homes filled with smoke from these stoves are a leading cause of infant and child mortality.

Even in the United States, indoor air pollution is more of a problem than outdoor air pollution. The U.S. Environmental Protection Agency recently ranked indoor air pollution as the fourth highest cancer risk among thirteen environmental factors. Levels of pollutants such as formaldehyde, styrene, xylene, and chloroform were two to fifty times higher indoors than outdoors.

Indoor air pollution also includes radon (the number one environmental cause of cancer); VOCs (volatile organic compounds) emitted by paints, lacquers, and solvents; secondhand tobacco smoke; carbon monoxide; the dry cleaning solvents TCE and PCE (trichloroethylene and perchloroethylene); and heavy metals such as lead, mercury, and arsenic.

A report by the California Air Resources Board found that indoor air pollution cost the state $45 billion in 2005 due to adult hospital and emergency room visits, lost productivity at work, and treatment for children suffering from asthma, allergies, and respiratory and heart disease.

Considering what you know now about the immune system, this should not come as a surprise. These diseases are related to immune activation, which is triggered by air pollution. Findings reported in the February 2006 *American Journal of Respiratory and Critical Care Medicine* showed that CRP levels rose significantly two days after people were exposed to air pollution.

Indoor air pollution can be a problem both at home and at work. Office buildings have been linked with a number of respiratory health problems. The term "sick building syndrome" (SBS) has been coined to describe buildings with excessive accumulation of noxious substances without adequate ventilation to help eliminate them. SBS can be dangerous to your immune system. The World Health Organization has suggested that up to 30 percent of new and remodeled buildings worldwide may be linked with SBS symptoms.

The keys to controlling indoor air pollution are ventilation and filtration.

Ventilation is crucial for buildings to breathe properly. Radon, for example, is a common, natural, radioactive gas that percolates up through the ground and gets trapped inside houses; it's much more of a problem in newer, more airtight, higher-efficiency homes because they tend to trap the gas inside. Older, leakier homes generally have fewer radon problems, because there's more air movement and cross-ventilation in them.

There's a common saying in medicine: "The solution to pollution is dilution." This applies whether you're talking about germs in an infected wound, a poisonous ingestion, or skin contact with some chemical. In the case of indoor air pollution, dilution equals ventilation. Keep the air moving. Unless you're living in an area with very high levels of outdoor air pollution, chances are your air quality indoors is worse than that outdoors. In most cases, good ventilation can help dilute indoor air pollution and reduce immune activation.

Filtration is another way to improve indoor air quality. High-volume air filters that screen out very small particles can be helpful in reducing particulate indoor air pollution. HEPA (high-efficiency particulate air) filters are now available for homes, vacuum cleaners, and even surgical operating rooms.

YOUR WORK ENVIRONMENT

If you work in a poorly ventilated or highly sealed building, one that is constructed with or houses many chemicals or artificial products, you could be working in a sick building. The tip-off is if you feel sick at work but fine at home, or if you find yourself feeling much better when you leave the office for extended periods of time. Not long ago one patient told me that he loved his vacations in the Rocky Mountains because it was the only time he felt truly healthy. We later discovered that he'd been suffering a reaction to the poor air quality in his office. Once that was dealt with by filtering the air with a high-volume HEPA filter, keeping his windows open, and adding several large, leafy plants to the office—such as ming aralia—he felt great, even at work.

The newest HEPA filters are capable of filtering out particles smaller than one micron (a micron is one millionth of a meter, or about 0.00003937 inches. That's small, as an average bacterium is about one to five microns in size.) A good HEPA filter can screen out more than 99 percent of airborne particles down to 0.3 microns.

HEPA filters are rated by their efficiency (how effectively they can screen out such small particles) and their volume (how big a space they can effectively filter). If particulate air pollution, allergies, asthma, or respiratory disorders are problems for you, consider a HEPA system big enough to filter your entire home. If not, there are room-sized units to filter the one or two rooms in which you spend the most time. When you change the filter, its filthiness will help you realize how dirty your indoor air is, and how much strain you just removed from your immune system.

CLEAN WATER

Besides pure air, your immune system also needs clean water. Yet most people assume their water is clean as long as it looks clear and uncolored and tastes okay.

Around the world, low water quality and poor sanitation are the principal cause of illness. According to the United Nations Children's Fund, 42 percent of the world's households lack a toilet, and one in six people do not have access to safe water. Thirty-five percent of the world has a drastic shortage of clean drinking water.

The World Health Organization recognizes 5 liters per day for cooking and drinking as the bare minimum per-person water requirement. For cleanliness and good health, about 30 liters per person per day are needed. Yet a billion people on earth have access to less than 5 liters of clean water per day.

In contrast, water usage in the United States is a whopping 700 liters per day per person. If you find this hard to believe, consider that an average bath uses 140 liters, and an average five-minute shower about 75 liters, or that each conventional toilet flush uses 19 liters (low-flush toilets use 5½).

With such a seemingly endless supply of clean water, Americans assume it is not a precious resource; just turn on the tap and out it flows.

But despite our easy access to tap water, truly clean water is hard to come by. A 2002 United States Geological Survey study of water samples from thirty states found that 80 percent of the streams, lakes, and rivers in the country were contaminated with chemicals, including contraceptives, painkillers, antibiotics, pesticides, caffeine, insect repellent, household cleaners, veterinary medicines, perfumes, and nicotine.

We know this because the government monitors our water supply. The EPA is responsible for setting national standards for pub-

---

RADON HOME TEST

Radon levels in the ground vary by location, but it's easy and inexpensive to test your home for radon gas. The Environmental Protection Agency (EPA) offers information on radon at www.epa.gov/radon, including which areas of the country have the highest levels. It also provides a link to state-by-state radon assistance contacts. Kits for testing home radon cost between ten and forty dollars and are often available at home and hardware stores. If you find you have a problem, eliminating radon requires improving ventilation so it can escape. Ask a local remediation specialist for advice tailored to your situation.

---

lic drinking water, and it maintains them for eighty-three different contaminants, including bacteria and other microorganisms, chlorine and bromine by-products, disinfectants, inorganic and organic chemicals, and radiation.

Not infrequently, municipalities flunk their water quality tests. One of the most publicized examples was the Washington, DC, water supply, which was found to have lead contamination in January 2004. This event made national news when it came to light that the DC Water and Sewer Authority knew of the lead contamination for more than a year and had not informed the public. After public disclosure was made, 3 percent of children voluntarily tested in the DC area had elevated blood lead levels.

CLEAN ENVIRONMENT

Frankly, our bodies have become toxic waste dumps. The Centers for Disease Control's Third National Report on Human Exposure to Chemicals, released in 2005, tested and found more than

140 contaminants in participants' bloodstreams. Although there has been improvement in regulations to reduce exposure to poisons including tobacco smoke, pesticides, and lead, the report showed continued widespread contamination with heavy metals including mercury and cadmium, and synthetic chemicals and by-products, such as plasticizers and dioxins.

These reports are disturbing because of the effect of pollution—

FILTER YOUR WATER

Home water filter systems can produce safe, healthy water that is often better than many varieties of bottled water. Several different kinds of filtration systems are available, and which you should use will depend on your local water quality and what contaminants your tap water might contain. To help you decide on the best water filter, get your water tested—you can find commercial testing companies online or in the phone book. One that I've used in the past is www. ULdrinkwell.com. If this service seems too expensive, use your local county water quality report (available at www.epa.gov/water/region .html) and advice from local water quality experts.

Here is a brief summary of the types of home water filtration systems available:

- **Pitchers/carafes:** Convenient and low in cost, these filtering pitchers are filled up with water from your tap. Most brands, such as the popular Brita water filter, use a combination filter made with activated charcoal and ion-exchange resin. These filters produce water with reduced chlorine and other bad tastes, as well as fewer sediments, but eliminate only some metals (lead, copper) and parasites (giardia, cryptosporidiosis). The pitchers do not remove chemicals such as VOCs, pesticides, or chloroform. Most carafes hold about ten cups.

---

exposure to a number of environmental toxins has been linked with autoimmune diseases.

Asbestos is another immune activator. Vermiculite miners in Libby, Montana, exposed to asbestos were found to have elevated levels of antinuclear antibodies (*Environmental Health Perspectives*, January 2005).

Mercury exposure has also been linked with subsequent

- **Faucet-mount systems:** Well-known brands such as PUR and Brita provide faucet-mounted filtration that filters water as it exits the tap, which makes them great for grabbing a quick glass of water or for making coffee or ice. The three-stage model is also designed to filter chloroform. Filters need to be changed every hundred gallons or so, and cost about fifteen dollars each.

- **Under-the-sink systems:** More discreet and robust, under-the-sink systems can last longer without a filter change (usually every six months or so). Results are similar to faucet-mount systems. These tend to be rather expensive.

- **Reverse-osmosis systems:** Reverse osmosis uses a series of thin membranes to purify water and produces the purest water available from home systems. This type of system requires a separate spigot for the purified water and is quite expensive. Some can be installed under sinks, but they can also be installed to treat the entire household's water. Their disadvantage is that they waste two to five gallons for every gallon of water filtered— not the best system in areas where water is scarce or expensive.

For more information on brands and the performance of various filtration systems, visit www.consumerreports.org.

---

development of autoimmune diseases in animals. Even low-level mercury exposure in mice led to an autoimmune kidney disease called glomerulonephritis (*Environmental Health Perspectives*, August 2003).

The point is that our immune system doesn't like exposure to unknown chemicals, which can affect it in many ways, and seldom for the better. Scientists are still learning how drugs and environmental toxins affect our immune system over the long term. The hope is that we may someday find better ways to manipulate our immune system to strengthen its ability to protect us without simultaneously causing autoimmunity and aging.

ALLERGENS AROUND THE HOUSE

When you alter your external environment in order to soothe the immune system, remember to eliminate the often invisible other inhabitants of your surroundings. Mold, mildew, and critters such as small insects and mites are a few of the local denizens that can wreak havoc with immunity.

MOLDS

Mold is one of the environmental pollutants most irritating to the immune system. And mold can grow almost anywhere, especially in dark, moist places. It can also cause strange and unusual symptoms that often elude even the most expert diagnostics. That's partly because there's no single blood test, scan, or skin test that can accurately and specifically diagnose a reaction to mold.

Molds commonly known to cause human disease include *Blastomyces, Coccidioides, Cryptococcus, Histoplasma, Candida,* and *Aspergillus.* Many more can cause serious illness in patients with compromised immunity. Diseases caused by molds can spread in unusual ways; for example, valley fever is caused by mold from soil blown around by the wind in southwestern states.

Homes harbor molds in dark, moist corners, especially in basements, bathrooms, and attics. Millions of dollars of real estate have been intentionally demolished by owners in last-ditch attempts to get rid of tenacious molds.

The most infamous of the toxic molds affecting homeowners is called *Stachybotrys*, or stachy for short. Stachy is a black mold often found in homes with drainage or moisture problems. Once it starts forming, it's extremely tough to get rid of. A tremendous amount of controversy exists as to what degree stachy is responsible for human illness. However, inhabitants of stachy-infected homes invariably complain of innumerable symptoms, from typical allergy symptoms to skin problems, arthritis, and autoimmune diseases.

We've occasionally had patients come in with chronic allergies and other conditions. In a number of instances, after testing for multiple causes, we finally suspected the illnesses came from exposure to mold, and the patients didn't improve until they eliminated the mold in their homes.

Nancy, for example, is a fifty-year-old accountant who suffered from chronic migraines. She had tried every cure under the sun, but nothing seemed to work. Having exhausted all possibilities, and becoming afraid that we would never be able to make her feel better, we began trying an increasing number of esoteric and alternative treatments.

Finally, a blood test revealed that Nancy had extremely high levels of antibodies to the black mold stachy. We then wondered if perhaps she had *Stachybotrys* in her home, so we suggested an environmental assessment. It came back negative.

Then Nancy pointed out that her symptoms were at their worst while she was at work. So we repeated the assessment in her office, and eureka! Her office tested positive for stachy cultures.

The solution was to install HEPA filters in her office, while her employer addressed the primary source of the mold exposure. It was the first time in years Nancy had felt relief from her migraines.

Normally, when you think about allergies, you picture stuffiness, congestion, coughing. But Nancy's only symptom was migraines. It took an environmental analysis by experts, and some rather eso-teric blood tests, to find the problem, but you, too, should suspect mold when allergy symptoms such as headaches or unusual skin rashes appear and there is a possible mold problem at home or at work.

COCKROACHES

Another unwelcome inhabitant sharing your space can also exert a powerful immune-activating effect: cockroaches. These creatures are among the oldest in the insect world; cockroach fossils go as far back as 300 million years (the oldest human fossils are a mere thirty-five thousand years old).

A large-scale 2005 study of asthma and allergies funded by the National Institute of Environmental Health Sciences and the National Institute of Allergy and Infectious Diseases found that exposure to cockroach droppings was an important cause of asthma symptoms in children susceptible to the cockroach allergen.

The study also found that the majority of homes in Chicago, Manhattan, and the Bronx had levels of cockroach allergens high enough to trigger symptoms. One in five people are allergic to the cockroach allergens found in cockroach dung.

Cockroach allergy seems to be caused by cytokines generated by the immune system, namely interleukin-8, which is released in the lungs, causing asthma.

Unfortunately, cockroaches can be tough to eradicate. Be sure to keep all food in sealed containers and stop dripping faucets. Some people have had good luck with what's commonly called a Las Vegas roach trap, which is simply an empty mayonnaise or pickle jar partially filled with coffee grounds and water and leaned against a wall for easier entry. The coffee grounds attract the roaches, and once in the jar they can't climb out and either drown or are trapped.

DUST MITES

Even if you manage to rid yourself of cockroaches, you should look out for something smaller and almost as bad for your immune system: dust mites. Thankfully, they aren't as allergenic as cockroaches, but they are more common. Dust mites are microscopic creatures that thrive in our homes, and are a common cause of asthma, allergies, skin rashes, and itchy eyes. They also activate our immune system.

House dust mites survive, not surprisingly, on dust, which is largely composed of shed human skin cells. The skin shed from a single person in just one day can feed a million dust mites!

Controlling dust mites requires controlling dust. Vacuum cleaners with HEPA filters are important. Wood or tile floors are preferable to carpeting because they're less likely to harbor dust and mites. Regular dusting is needed, as is reducing humidity in the house via a dehumidifier. Also, many mattress and pillow casings are available that reduce exposure to mites while you sleep.

TAKE ACTION: SOOTHE

We've already talked about the many steps you can take to make your environment as soothing as possible for your immune system. Still, there's always more to do, because the world is not a soothing place. Any way you can find to make your immediate environment a happier one, do it—your immune system will be grateful. Here are some reminders.

1. **Inspect your home for potential allergens:** Examine corners in bathrooms and basements for standing water. Fix any leaks

in ceilings or roofs. Check around ceiling fans in bathrooms for water stains. Look for black or greenish discoloration in any damp areas. Vacuum regularly with a HEPA-equipped vacuum cleaner. Have your carpeting cleaned professionally, or consider removing it and switching to wood or cork flooring. Put out a few Las Vegas–style roach traps along the baseboard of your kitchen for a few nights to see if you catch any roaches. Install a HEPA air cleaner in whichever rooms you use the most. Repair any leaking or dripping faucets or plumbing.

Also, consider a professional environmental analysis if you or others in your family are having allergic or unusual symptoms that elude a diagnosis.

2. **Make your home a peaceful oasis:** Hang your favorite pictures. Fill vases with fresh flowers. Display your favorite artwork. Disregard fashion trends and use colors and styles you love to create an eclectic and comfortable blend of furnishings and decorations. Create a central place in the kitchen, dining area, or family room for congregating with friends and family. Let sunlight stream in during the day. Place candles about to generate a warm feeling in the evening. Light a fire in the fireplace during the winter months. Play your favorite music all day long. Fill your place with wonderful smells such as fresh flowers, jasmine, home-baked bread, or mulled apple cider.

3. **Do a home walk-through:** Make a to-do list of any areas that need attention, especially noting any water stains, trapped moisture, condensation, bubbled paint or drywall, and any visible mold. Have your carpets cleaned professionally. (Leave the house while they're being cleaned.) Steam clean your upholstery once a year. Launder spreads, throws, and blankets. Vacuum regularly with a HEPA-equipped vacuum.

4. **Have your water tested:** Choose a water filter that addresses any contaminants you discover, or, if you find none, consider a simple filtered carafe or pitcher.

5. **Take care of your air:** Consider a HEPA filter for your bedroom or family room to reduce any particulate air pollution, and a central air filter system if your home is dusty.

6. **Schedule weekly time with your partner for sharing massages:** Use fragrant aromatherapy oils to your taste. If you don't have a partner, consider making an appointment with a masseur or masseuse for a professional massage. You can also purchase simple and inexpensive equipment that will help you to massage yourself; there are many varieties on the market, from vibrating thumpers or chairs to simple back-scratcher units that allow you to apply pressure to the muscles around your spine, neck, and shoulders. Don't forget to massage your own feet by hand.

7. **Take a warm bath:** Light some candles. Add some aromatherapeutic drops.

8. **Make music:** Turn on your radio, portable music, or CD player. If you can, play music—piano, flute, guitar. If you can't play an instrument, then sing. If you can't sing, then hum!

9. **Mask unwanted noise:** If you live on a noisy street, add some soothing background sounds, such as a water feature that trickles over rocks or a vertical wall. Surprisingly inexpensive, these are available in many catalogs or online.

10. **Turn off your phone:** Not permanently—just for an hour or two now and then to eliminate intrusion into your peaceful

space. Especially important times to do this are during dinner, or when you're recharging in your bathtub, having or giving a massage, or making love. The same goes for pagers, Black-Berries, instant messaging, and e-mail.

11. **Put your feet up:** By the end of the day, they're as tired as you are. In fact, put your legs and your hips up too. If you have sore feet, swollen ankles, or a bad back, inverting your body can be soothing. Try lying down on an inclined ramp, or using an inversion table (available online) for twenty minutes a day. It's easy to make an inclined ramp at home using a couple of two-by-six or two-by-eight boards, a sturdy stool or chair, and a few blankets.

12. **Consider getting an aquarium:** Make it a Zen experience—create an aquatic environment with the same enthusiasm and energy you put into your home.

13. **Create a getaway room:** If you have the space, designate one room in your house as a meditation or getaway room. This is a good place for that little waterfall, and for art, photographs, or other items that fill you with contentment. Many people find that such a room puts them in a happier state of mind the moment they enter it.

14. **Come up with your own ideas:** Paint your bedroom a soothing color. Hang a wind chime on your back porch. If there's something that will make you feel more relaxed, at ease, and at home, then do it!

STEP 7: ENHANCE

IN THE SOOTHE step, you learned how to quiet an aggravated immune system by changing your external environment. Likewise, the immune system feels more secure, and is less likely to be activated, when you've optimized the performance of your internal environment.

Medical research has now proven that certain vitamins and nutritional supplements can enhance immune function and help to deactivate an overstimulated immune system—and not only keep you looking younger but actually keep you from aging too fast. Below are some of the key supplements. I can't imagine that anyone will want, or need, to take all these, but read on to find out what might work best for you and what should be taken by everyone.

SUPPLEMENTS

FISH OILS

Fish oils, also known as omega-3 oils, have been studied intensively over the last decade. The two most familiar are EPA and DHA (eicosapentaenoic acid and docosahexaenoic acid).

We talked about fish in the Eat step. But for those who simply don't like or don't eat enough fish, the alternative is taking purified fish oils in capsule form. This option is a much better one than in the old days, when your grandmother forced you to swallow unpleasant-tasting cod-liver oil.

Research shows that the higher someone's blood levels of fish oils, the lower the level of immune activation.

These days you must be careful about consuming fish and fish products because of contamination by heavy metals (such as mercury) and industrial chemicals (such as polychlorinated biphenyls, or PCBs). Getting the right amount of fish oil without exposing yourself to unwanted contaminants can be difficult.

So when you're shopping, make sure you buy a high-quality fish oil, free of the contaminants found in the fish themselves. Look for information from the manufacturer that attests to its purity. For example, choose fish oil labeled "distilled," meaning that impurities and contaminants have been extracted, or pharmaceutical-grade fish oil, which must pass higher standards of quality and purity. Also, search out a USP label, which stands for United States Pharmacopeia, again meaning a higher standard has been used in the manufacture.

Personally, I prefer supplements from companies whose products have been tested for purity by independent labs, as advertised on their products. These companies contract with the labs to buy their vitamins or supplements off the shelf on an annual basis, test them in their own facilities, and publish the results.

Several consumer organizations also perform tests, including ConsumerLab.com, which buys fish oil and other vitamin products, tests them for purity, and compares their results with the information on the product's own label. It then provides a rating showing how well the vitamin or fish oil under study lives up to its own claims.

The proper fish oil dose varies by individual, but I usually recommend one to three grams per day. If you're taking fish oil simply to prevent immune activation, you can use less—about one gram (1,000 milligrams) a day, which is usually the amount found in one or two high-potency capsules.

MULTIVITAMINS

Multivitamins contain a mixture of all the vitamins A through E and vitamin K, plus essential minerals.

For years doctors have been recommending that people take vitamin supplements; however, surveys consistently show that only two in five Americans actually do so. This is unfortunate, because in addition to their other positive effects, multivitamins have been scientifically shown to lower CRP levels after just six months of use (*American Journal of Medicine*, December 15, 2003).

The same recommendations for choosing a high-quality fish oil apply when searching for a multivitamin. Find one from a reputable manufacturer who certifies the quality of its product, and that has either been lab tested or carries the USP label. Ideally, your multivitamin should contain only vitamins and nutrients, without unnecessary fillers, colorings, preservatives, stabilizers, or glaze.

Just about everybody should be taking a multivitamin, but it's especially important for certain people, such as children, who, being picky eaters, tend to avoid nutrient-rich foods, and pregnant women, who should look for special prenatal multivitamins.

Not only do people who take a daily multivitamin enjoy lower CRP levels; research shows that they have enhanced immune function and come down with fewer colds and respiratory infections. They also miss fewer days of work—all of which means that they age better than those who don't take multivitamins.

VITAMIN D

Vitamin D is often called the sunshine vitamin. Technically speaking, it's not really a vitamin at all, but a hormone that our bodies manufacture when exposed to sunlight. And indeed, there was a time when people got as much vitamin D as they needed by being outdoors.

But today, when people spend more time indoors than ever before—and slather themselves with sunblock when they do go out, thanks to constant warnings about the damage sun can do to the skin—that's no longer the case. Applying sunblock is an excellent way to avoid the harm that can lead to skin cancer, but it also impedes needed ultraviolet light from reaching our skin, where vitamin D is produced. So in the process of protecting our skin, we're also reducing our odds of getting sufficient vitamin D.

Indeed, recent studies show that nearly everyone who lives in a temperate climate is vitamin D deficient, as are approximately 1 billion people worldwide.

Low levels of vitamin D have been linked with significant immunological disorders, including multiple sclerosis, the nerve disorder that leads to loss of function and paralysis. It's long been known that while multiple sclerosis is common in temperate climates, few cases are reported around the equator. We don't know exactly why, but the new thinking is that the difference is vitamin D related.

Vitamin D deficiency has also been linked with osteoporosis, depression, obesity, heart disease, inflammatory bowel disease, and at least a dozen forms of cancer, including breast and prostate cancer, as well as autoimmune disorders such as type 1 diabetes and arthritis.

Food sources of vitamin D include fortified products into which vitamin D has been added, such as milk, yogurt, and other dairy products; cereals; and soymilk. Fatty fish also provide vitamin D; for example, four ounces of salmon contains about 400 IU (10 micrograms) of vitamin D; about the same amount is found in sardines, mackerel, and canned tuna (choose the chunk-light variety, which is lowest in contaminants).

All daily multivitamins contain at least some vitamin D, ranging from a low of 100 units to about 400 units. But most people who live in temperature climates should take more than 400 units daily.

It takes about twenty minutes of daily sun exposure on the face and arms—or any other similarly sized body parts—to produce your requirement for vitamin D. But since we all take in vitamin D somewhat differently, and too much sun can cause skin damage and cancer, the solution is vitamin D supplements.

When shopping for a vitamin D supplement, realize that there are actually five different forms of vitamin D (vitamin D1, D2, D3, etc.), and they go by different names, such as ergocalciferol and cholecalciferol.

Vitamin D3 (cholecalciferol) is most effective. Research suggests that optimal intake of vitamin D3 is 800 to 1,000 IU (20 to 25 micrograms) per day. Some people need even higher levels, depending on their absorption of the vitamin, their genetics, and their medical condition, so it's best to measure and monitor levels of vitamin D through blood tests. Ask your doctor at your next physical.

When doctors test your blood, they are looking for the level of what's known as 25-hydroxy vitamin D, which should be well over 40, with optimal levels between 75 nmol/L (nanomoles per liter) and 100 nmol/L.

Warning: It is possible to overdose on vitamin D, but usually at levels only over 10,000 IU daily, which is far more than you could absorb from any supplement (when taken as directed) combined with diet and exposure to sunshine.

VITAMINS C AND E

Scientists have long known about the value of taking extra vitamin C, in great part because of the experiments undertaken in the 1960s and 1970s by Nobel laureate Dr. Linus Pauling, who believed people were not ingesting anything close to their actual vitamin C requirements; he recommended a daily dose as high as 3,000 to 6,000 milligrams. Pauling's research interested many others in studying vitamin C, but later studies didn't corroborate a need for such sizable doses.

When interest in vitamin C waned, vitamin E picked up the

slack. It, too, was then considered a wonder drug, but like vitamin C, it failed to live up to initial claims.

Interestingly, recent research shows that these two vitamins work best in tandem rather than individually. Taken together, vitamins C and E seem to have a powerful effect on the immune system. Tests on people who take the two in combination show low CRP levels and less immune activation. However, the amounts of C and E needed to achieve these effects exceed what is usually present in the average multivitamin. So I generally recommend taking about 250 to 500 milligrams of vitamin C, and 100 to 400 IUs a day of vitamin E, in addition to your multivitamin.

Vitamin C is found in many foods, particularly citrus fruits and vegetables such as tomatoes, potatoes, and broccoli. It's easily manufactured, fairly stable, and at the recommended dosages has few if any side effects. Because synthetic vitamin C is identical to naturally occurring vitamin C—there are no known differences in their actions or absorption—it's fine to buy generic vitamin C.

You should be a little choosier when shopping for vitamin E, however. The most commonly used form of vitamin E in typical mass-market vitamins is dl-alpha tocopherol, a synthetic form that is hard for humans to absorb. A better form is known as mixed natural tocopherols, which contains naturally occurring forms of vitamin E including alpha, beta, gamma, and delta tocopherols.

Some research suggests that gamma tocopherol may be more important in the prevention of health problems than the more commonly available alpha tocopherol. In fact, taking too much of the alpha type depletes levels of gamma tocopherol, which might explain the recent flurry of research failing to show benefits from taking vitamin E. In these studies, only the alpha tocopherol was given.

B VITAMINS

B vitamins seem to have a powerful effect on the immune system. One of the most important is vitamin B6, or pyridoxine, which is found in many foods, including meats, fish, nuts, beans, grains, and some fruits. Low levels of vitamin B6 in the blood have been associated with higher CRP levels (as noted in an article in the June 2001 *Journal of Circulation*).

Most people should take about 50 to 100 milligrams of B6 a day. Check your multivitamin to see if it contains that amount; if it doesn't, consider looking for a higher-quality multivitamin.

Be careful, however: an overdose of B6 can be dangerous, causing loss of balance (ataxia), neuropathy (nerve damage), and skin rashes. It's best not to exceed 100 milligrams daily.

Another of the B vitamins is vitamin B12, also known as cobalamin, which works in concert with vitamin B6. Vitamin B12 is unique among vitamins in that it isn't found in the plant world; it's only made in the animal kingdom, so vegans must use B12 supplements.

Vitamin B12 deficiency has been linked with dementia, nerve damage, numbness, and loss of balance. Vitamin B12 is also necessary for maintaining proper levels of homocysteine (high homocysteine levels have been linked with heart disease, dementia, Alzheimer's disease, stroke, diabetes, and cancer).

Signs of deficiency include a smooth, shiny, and glossy tongue that lacks the usual tiny bumps and brushlike surface.

Good dietary sources of vitamin B12 include meat, dairy products, eggs, and shellfish. Cereal products are commonly fortified with vitamin B12, and yeasts are also capable of producing it.

The usual recommendation is 0.5 milligram to 1 milligram a day. Your multivitamin may already contain that much, in which case you don't need to take more. But if it doesn't, you should add it to your daily regime.

SELENIUM

Minerals, too, can help reduce immune activation and lower CRP levels. One of these is selenium, an important trace element found in foods such as Brazil nuts, beef, and chicken breast. However, selenium deficiency can occur in geographic areas where soils are depleted and animal feed is low in the nutrient.

Low selenium levels have been linked with heart attacks, cancer, and a number of diseases of immune activation. In fact, selenium depletion seems to occur whenever CRP production increases—that is, blood levels of selenium are found to drop significantly when CRP levels rise. Low selenium levels have also been shown to be associated with higher levels of the immune-activating cytokine interleukin-6.

Selenium supplements can help to lower CRP levels in people with some autoimmune diseases, such as psoriasis (an autoimmune skin disorder). However, selenium toxicity can occur if supplementation is excessive, causing hair loss, brittle nails, skin rash, garliclike breath odor, and fatigue.

Selenium supplementation safely ranges from 50 to 200 micrograms per day. Caution is advised in eating Brazil nuts, as one ounce (about six to eight nuts) can contain as much as 500 to 800 micrograms of selenium. A good rule is that each fresh (shelled) Brazil nut contains about 100 micrograms of selenium. If you are supplementing with selenium, it's advisable not to eat more than a couple Brazil nuts a day.

ZINC

Zinc is a critical component of thousands of proteins in the body and plays an especially important role in immunity, a fact of which most people have become aware due to the recent popularity of zinc lozenges for treating the common cold.

Rich dietary sources of zinc include oysters, beef, and chicken. Peas, beans, legumes, and almonds are reasonable vegetarian sources.

Adults need between 10 and 40 milligrams of zinc per day. Signs of zinc deficiency include hair loss, diarrhea, fatigue, and slow wound healing. In men, zinc is concentrated in the prostate, and semen contains one hundred times as much zinc as the blood, so men who are very sexually active require more than the usual amount of zinc. In addition, in both men and women, caffeine, calcium, iron, and phosphorus can block zinc absorption.

Zinc deficiency is common among alcoholics; about one-third to one-half of alcoholics are zinc deficient. Deficiency also occurs with chronic diarrhea, digestive disorders, and malabsorption, and is more common among vegetarians because zinc from vegetable sources is not absorbed well.

Zinc deficiency is also more common in the elderly, who absorb it less efficiently, and this results in immune activation and progressively higher levels of TNF-alpha, interleukin-6, and other immune-activating cytokines.

In fact, zinc depletion may be a common cause of the immune activation that occurs as we age. It has been reported that zinc deficiency is present in about 20 percent of young and middle-aged adults, but is present in as many as 63 percent of nonagenarians (90-year-olds).

The recommended supplemental dose to assure adequate zinc levels is 10 to 20 milligrams daily. People with special needs (such as the elderly and those with digestive disorders, inflammatory conditions, or who drink alcohol in excess) should be taking higher doses.

But too much zinc can also cause problems; daily intakes of hundreds of milligrams can deplete the body of copper and impair immune function.

MAGNESIUM

Magnesium is a vital mineral, important for nerve, bone, and muscle function, as well as for the regulation of heart rhythm. We require between 400 and 600 milligrams of magnesium per day. Unfortunately, low magnesium is common—most Americans get less than 300 milligrams daily. Magnesium deficiency has been linked with high blood pressure, asthma, migraine, constipation, osteoporosis, diabetes, heart arrhythmias, and cancer. It has been found in one-third of nursing home residents and about two-thirds of seriously ill patients in intensive care units, and in substantial numbers of otherwise healthy adults. About 10 to 15 percent of the general population, and as many as one in five young urban African American women, are thought to be seriously deficient. Despite this, no mineral deficiency is more underdiagnosed than magnesium deficiency.

Conditions that require extra magnesium include alcoholism; chronic diarrhea and gastrointestinal problems that cause malabsorption; chronic, excessive stress; and diabetes.

Food sources rich in magnesium include green leafy vegetables, whole grains, nuts, legumes (beans and peas), apricots, and soy foods.

Magnesium supplementation can enhance immune function, especially in cases of immune activation. A variety of types of magnesium supplements are available, but the best tolerated and absorbed are probably magnesium glycinate or other amino acid chelates. These supplements are best taken with food and spread out in divided doses over the day, with meals. For example, you might take 120 milligrams of magnesium glycinate with each meal.

(Too much magnesium, however, causes diarrhea and stomach cramps, but it's hard to overdose on oral magnesium except when kidney function is impaired, as is the case in dialysis patients.)

GLUTATHIONE

In addition to vitamins and minerals, several nonvitamin supplements can help enhance our immune function, including small proteins or amino acids, the building blocks of proteins.

One of the most important small proteins is glutathione, three amino acids in length. Glutathione, made by the body, plays an important role in many chemical processes within our system, especially detoxification. Glutathione also has an anti-inflammatory effect on the immune system and is known to ameliorate immune activation.

Unfortunately, glutathione may not be absorbed well when taken orally. The body can be encouraged to manufacture glutathione, however, if it has enough of the proper building blocks in place. Some of these building blocks come from the cruciferous vegetable family, which includes broccoli, cauliflower, cabbage, kale, bok choy, and brussels sprouts. By eating more of those vegetables, you'll make more glutathione.

Glutathione is available as a supplement, however; called reduced glutathione, it can be dissolved in the mouth rather than swallowed, allowing more glutathione to be absorbed through the cheeks and gums. Take 100 to 200 milligrams per day.

NAC

N-acetyl cysteine, or NAC, is an amino acid that works by boosting levels of glutathione, and in turn helps to reduce immune activation. Doctors use NAC to treat poisonings and overdoses of, for example, Tylenol (acetaminophen) and to protect patients from X-ray dyes. Because NAC is an amino acid, it can be taken orally and is well absorbed. N-acetyl cysteine works well in combination with another supplement known as L-carnitine.

One to three grams a day is generally safe, but too much can be a problem for some people, who may form cysteine kidney stones. It's not found in this form in foods, but the broccoli family has cysteine analogues.

L-CARNITINE

L-carnitine is a natural amino acid–like compound that can enhance immune function and has been given to kidney dialysis patients to lower their CRP levels. It is usually taken in doses between 2,000 and 4,000 milligrams per day.

Another form of carnitine, known as acetyl-L-carnitine, may be absorbed more readily, allowing for lower doses, between 500 and 1,500 milligrams per day.

L-ARGININE

L-arginine is another important amino acid that reduces immune activation. It is especially helpful to people with high blood pressure and men who suffer from erectile dysfunction; L-arginine seems to have an effect similar to medicines such as Viagra.

L-arginine has also been used to treat a variety of conditions, from heart failure to pituitary gland disorders to migraine headaches. Dosage of L-arginine is usually between 1,500 and 6,000 milligrams per day.

Caution should be taken under certain circumstances, such as if you suffer from asthma; L-arginine may aggravate symptoms. Similarly, L-arginine may pose some danger if given immediately after a heart attack.

QUERCETIN

Quercetin is one of a group of compounds known as flavonoids which also includes citrus compounds such as naringin, rutin, and hesperidin, among others. It is found in such diverse foods as apples, tea, onions, and broccoli. Quercetin and other flavonoids exhibit anti-inflammatory and immune-enhancing properties. Quercetin is usually taken in doses of 500 milligrams once or twice daily.

LIPOIC ACID

This supplement is a naturally occurring sulfur-based compound also known as alpha-lipoic acid or thioctic acid; it is found in spinach, broccoli, brewer's yeast, and red meat. Our bodies use lipoic acid as a catalyst for chemical reactions involving energy production and for boosting the production of glutathione. Supplements of lipoic acid are fairly well absorbed from capsules and may be helpful in treating autoimmune disorders such as diabetes and multiple sclerosis, and degenerative brain disorders.

A German study of lipoic acid given to mice in combination with the prescription medication selegiline (deprenyl) produced mice that lived twice as long as control animals.

Lipoic acid is found naturally in foods such as leafy green vegetables, beef, brewer's yeast, and tomatoes.

CHROMIUM PICOLINATE

As mentioned, carrying around too much weight can be a fundamental trigger for immune activation. After all, extra weight means extra fat. Extra fat produces extra immune-activating cytokines, including leptin. When we lose fat, leptin levels decrease and so does immune activation.

It's especially important to eliminate the type of fat carried around the middle, inside the belly, in the abdominal cavity. This particular type of fat produces more leptin than any other, and is more likely to cause activation of the immune system than the fat around your hips, under your skin, or on the back of your arms.

Chromium picolinate is one of the supplements that can help reverse the accumulation of body fat. Chromium is known for its ability to help promote weight loss and regulate blood sugar levels, especially in diabetic patients. Scientific research has shown that chromium picolinate helps type 2 diabetics lose weight and improve blood sugar readings when taken at a dose of 400 to 1,000 micrograms daily for four to six months.

The action of chromium picolinate in promoting weight loss and blood sugar regulation is due in part to its effect on the immune system, as it inhibits the release of the immune-activating cytokines TNF-alpha and interleukin-6 from white blood cells.

In fact, cytokines play an important role in the vicious circle that so many people experience of weight loss followed by weight gain. The rebound weight gain that tends to occur after you struggle to lose weight is triggered by an increase in cytokines, putting you right back where you started—but even more frustrated and despondent.

Chromium can be found in brewer's yeast, as well as in beef, liver, eggs, chicken, oysters, wheat germ, apples, bananas, and spinach. For purposes of helping to control blood sugar and improve insulin sensitivity, dosages of 400 to 500 micrograms per day are used.

In addition to chromium picolinate, another readily available form of chromium is chromium polynicotinate. Dosages of up to 1,000 micrograms for up to six months appear to be safe, although scientific data on the long-term safety of high-dose chromium are still lacking.

Fiber

Another important, and often neglected, supplement is fiber. Research indicates an inverse relationship between fiber and immune activation—the higher the fiber intake, the lower the immune activation.

Fiber is important for many reasons, from its ability to improve bowel function to its role in weight loss. People who consume a high-fiber diet tend to feel full sooner and are less apt to overeat.

Probably the most important effect of fiber is in promoting the growth of healthy bacteria in the gut, which in turn helps protect us from more dangerous and invasive bacteria. As discussed, the digestive tract is a pivotal location in terms of our body's homeland security. Creating a peaceful and nonthreatening environment in the gut is critical for maintaining peace throughout the immune system—it's impossible to have a relaxed immune system if the gut is continually triggering an immune response.

Beneficial, symbiotic bacteria such as lactobacilli and bifidobacteria feed on fiber and will thrive in an environment that provides them with enough food, just as we do when we consume enough food. Unlike humans, who lack the ability to digest fiber, these bacteria derive their energy from eating our undigested fiber.

When symbiotic bacteria flourish in our gut, their sheer numbers crowd out the unwanted and dangerous bacteria that compete for the same food. Thus to promote the growth and tip the balance in favor of healthy bacteria, we need to maintain an adequate intake of fiber.

Fiber can be easily obtained in the diet, from vegetables, fruits, and whole grains, but many types of supplements are also available. Your goal should be about 20 grams of fiber a day for every 1,000 calories you eat. So if you are consuming 1,500 calories a day, you need about 30 grams of fiber daily, either in your diet or by taking a supplement. You can also combine the two. If you're getting 15 fiber grams in your meals, you might want to add another 15 via supplement.

Common fiber supplements include psyllium husks (found in such brands as Konsyl), methylcellulose (found in Citrucel), and guar gum (found in Benefiber). Look for fiber supplements that are all natural and have no preservatives, fillers, or inactive or artificial ingredients. For example, you can try Metagenics's Herbulk or MetaFiber, or ProThera's SpectraFiber, which are blends of different sources of natural fiber.

To avoid constipation, drink eight glasses of water daily along with your fiber supplements.

WATER

Although water is not technically a supplement, its importance is impossible to overestimate here. Too often, people rely on thirst as a cue for when they need to drink. However, thirst doesn't kick in until you've become about 2 percent dehydrated. For a 180-pound person, that amounts to a loss of about three and a half pounds of body weight!

Fluid requirements for the average adult are about sixty-four ounces (two quarts) per day, which will generally come from bever-ages (ideally from clean, filtered water), and from water-rich foods such as fruits and vegetables.

Keep yourself constantly hydrated, and don't wait for thirst to trigger drinking. Keep a bottle of water nearby to remind you to drink more often—about eight glasses of water a day should suf-fice. I like adding a wedge or two of lemon or lime, which not only improves the taste but also adds limonene, a natural plant flavonoid calming to the immune system.

Rather than keeping track of ounces of fluid you're getting each day, use your urine as a guide. If you're urinating clear or pale yel-low every two hours or so, you are probably doing a good job with hydration. Dark, concentrated urine, or going four or more hours without urinating, usually means you need more fluid.

CHRONIC INFECTIONS

A lack of nutrients, fiber, or hydration is not the only reason behind activation of our internal environment. Remember that our immune system has evolved to respond to a real or perceived threat, and that threat is often the result of a lurking infection. Thus, one of the most important factors in helping your immune system to function properly is to make sure you have no hidden infections.

DANGER SIGNS

Most people associate an infection with symptoms such as a fever, cough, pain, boil, or some other tangible sign. The truth is that many people have chronic infections but don't know it because the infection may not be causing obvious symptoms. For example, a common stomach infection is caused by the bacterium *H. pylori*. *H. pylori* affects about 10 to 20 percent of Americans (and many more people in developing countries).

This particular bacterium has an unusual trait. Generally, when you swallow a germ, it quickly dies because the stomach is so acidic. This ability to kill germs is one of your stomach acid's most important qualities. But *H. pylori* actually thrives on acid; in fact, it can survive only in an acidic environment.

H. pylori was first discovered in 1892 in Italy, but it wasn't until 1992 that it was recognized as the cause of many stomach disorders, such as ulcers and cancer. It has also been found to cause gastritis and even eye problems such as blepharitis, or redness of the eyelid, and, as in our patient Cynthia (page 53), uveitis. And it's been linked with iron deficiency and skin disorders such as rosacea, a blotchy red face rash.

Other examples of chronic infections requiring treatment include (for men) prostate infections such as prostatitis. Because the prostate gland is buried between the bladder and the skin, it doesn't show obvious symptoms. But prostatitis eventually affects more than half of all men, and more than 60 percent of men over forty years old.

Chronic sinus infections now affect about 10 percent of Americans. Lyme disease can be found in half the people who live in endemic areas such as Martha's Vineyard or Nantucket, Massachusetts. Nationally, chlamydia is also common. People generally think of it as a sexually transmitted disease, but another species of chlamydia (*pneumoniae*) is a very common cause of bronchitis.

Many other conditions might be infectious diseases that we simply haven't recognized as such. Some of them have only recently been identified, such as Whipple's disease, an unusual bowel ailment causing malabsorption that can also lead to arthritis and problems with the heart, eyes, lungs, and brain. Whipple's disease was discovered in 1907, but the bacterium that causes it wasn't discovered until 1992.

Similarly, cat scratch fever, a fairly uncommon but serious infection resulting from a cat scratch, was first described in 1889, but the causative agent (a bacterium called *Bartonella henselae*) was not identified until 1988.

Even garden-variety arthritis may yet turn out to be an infectious disease.

If you are able to identify, treat, and eradicate these unsuspected infections, you can enhance your immune system and allow it to deactivate so it's no longer fighting germs all the time. Testing for such infections, however, can be challenging. It would be excellent if there were a single exam to check for all possible infections, but there isn't. Each one must be tested for individually, so the blood work you should have will depend on the most likely culprits. If you're living in Connecticut and have arthritis, you might want to be tested for Lyme disease. If you're always stuffed up with a runny nose or bronchitis, you probably should be tested for chlamydia. If you're a man and have urinary symptoms, you should check for prostatitis. If you have acid indigestion, heartburn, or gastritis, you should be tested for *H. pylori*.

Treating Infections with Probiotics

What can you do to treat a chronic infection? Even the most indolent infections leave some clues if they are of any significance to your immune system. For example, your white blood count may be elevated, your CRP may run high for no other reason, your urine sample may be abnormal, or you may have a chronic cough or digestive problems—all clues in tracking down otherwise unsuspected infections.

Many patients are tempted to take a course of antibiotics as a kind of shotgun treatment if they run into signs of immune activation due to infection. For some people, this might be worthwhile. But antibiotics are certainly not right for most people, because, as we know, they have serious side effects. Kids who have taken antibiotics develop more problems with allergies and asthma than those who haven't; women who've taken them seem to be at higher risk for breast cancer than those who haven't.

So antibiotics are not an innocuous treatment. They must be prescribed and used very carefully. In fact, antibiotics tend to be vastly overprescribed and even given for conditions not likely to respond to them, such as viral infections.

If you have an activated immune system and no other explanation can account for it, you may be well advised to take a course of antibiotics. This decision needs to be made deliberately by you and your physician.

Another type of supplement, called a probiotic, can help fight infection. While an antibiotic kills any and all bacteria, a probiotic promotes the growth of beneficial bacteria which, as we have seen, can compete with and crowd out undesirable bacteria in your system.

Probiotics, many of which can be found in foods such as yogurt, include acidophilus (*Lactobacillus acidophilus*), bifidobacteria, and/or some of the soil microorganisms.

Normally people have large quantities of these bacteria already inhabiting the lining of their gastrointestinal tract. However, many things can disrupt these levels. For example, stress shifts the balance of healthy bacteria toward the proliferation of undesirable and unwanted bacteria. So does a poor diet—or a course of antibiotics, which can indiscriminately kill bacteria, including the healthy kind.

The antidote to these immune activators is to take supplements of healthy probiotic bacteria, which help to shift the bacterial balance back in your favor. These supplements have been found successful in curing all sorts of infectious conditions, from diarrhea and ear infections to sinusitis and bronchitis.

Several tests can determine if you have enough friendly bacteria: stool cultures, urine tests, and breath tests.

When taking probiotics, look for high-potency brands that

supply at least 3 to 5 billion beneficial bacteria per dose. They should be taken for about four to six weeks at a time, especially during periods of stress or after a course of antibiotics.

PHYTONUTRIENTS

Phytonutrient supplements can enhance immune function and ameliorate immune activation. *Phyto,* which means "plant" in Greek, describes chemicals found in plants that have health benefits in humans. Many of the compounds that protect plants from disease, infection, or oxidation—and impart color and flavor—also have beneficial health effects in people. Science is continually discovering and testing new phytonutrients to uncover the secrets of their health effects. Here are some examples.

Silymarin: An active ingredient of the milk thistle plant, silymarin has been used as an herbal remedy for chronic hepatitis and cirrhosis. By helping to reduce the immune activation that occurs with these chronic diseases, silymarin may prevent the collateral damage to the liver that results from immune hyperactivity. Common dosages range between 160 and 480 milligrams daily.

Curcuminoids: Derived from turmeric root, and found in the same spice commonly used in curries, curcuminoids are also commonly used as a supplement for inflammatory and autoimmune conditions. Turmeric powder is the best source of curcumin for cooking in curries, and curcumin capsules are also available as supplements. Turmeric extracts are standardized at 90 to 95 percent curcumin, with dosages of 250 to 500 milligrams three times daily as needed.

Genistein: An isoflavone derived from soy, genistein blocks immune activation when taken in a dose of 10 to 20 milligrams per day. Genistein, which can be obtained from soy foods like tofu, tempeh, soymilk, and miso soup, is also available as an extract in capsule form.

Resveratrol: This phytonutrient, or plant compound, is found in the skin of grapes and in red wine, blueberries, and peanuts. (Resveratrol may be the source of some of the health benefits observed in cultures where wine is consumed with meals.) It is immune deactivating, anti-angiogenic, and seems to help prevent cancer, heart disease, and diabetes. Resveratrol is also available as a dietary supplement, at a dose of about 200 milligrams per day.

Polyphenols: These are a group of compounds common to many plants; they are responsible, for example, for the color of leaves as they change in autumn.

Teas are a good source of polyphenols, but these compounds are also found in peanuts, pomegranates, the skin of most fruits, dark chocolate, coffee, and extra virgin olive oil. Plant polyphenols have anticancer effects and protect against autoimmune disorders as well as aging. Some of the best ways to get your polyphenols are by drinking three cups of green tea daily, or one mug of dark coffee (decaf is okay), or by eating two to three ounces of dark chocolate. Red wine—in moderation!—is also a source.

Lycopene: This phytonutrient is found in tomatoes (especially cooked tomatoes) and other red vegetables, and can play a role in ameliorating inflammatory and autoimmune disorders. (Lycopene is available in many supplements, with dosages around 20 to 40 milligrams per day.)

Scientific research is continuing to add to the encyclopedia of immune-enhancing compounds on an almost daily basis. These substances will give us powerful tools to control our health by enhancing the function of our immune system.

MEDICATIONS

Common over-the-counter and prescription medications can also be used to alter our internal environment to enhance immune system function.

The very simplest of these is aspirin, which historically has been used to reduce fever because it blocks the immune system's production of pyrogens, cytokines that trigger a fever. Aspirin also lowers CRP levels, which is one reason it's used as a preventive for conditions such as heart attack and stroke.

Some interesting research suggests that aspirin might have even wider-ranging immune-boosting effects, including blocking the development of cancer and serving as an anti-angiogenic. It's also been shown to reduce the risk of colon cancer and the growth of colon polyps. So despite being simple and inexpensive, aspirin is extremely effective.

Some of the newer, more expensive—but not necessarily more effective—drugs to modulate the internal environment and the immune system include statin medications such as Lipitor, Zocor, and Pravachol. These medicines rose to fame because of their ability to lower cholesterol. But it seems they also reduce immune system activity and can effectively lower levels of C-reactive protein. In fact, studies have shown that it's reasonable to treat someone with a high CRP level with Lipitor or one of the other statins even if his or her cholesterol is normal.

However, like antibiotics, statins are not for everyone. They can have uncommon but serious side effects, including liver problems, muscle and nerve injury, and even amnesia. So be wary and talk to your doctor.

Even more powerful drugs are available to reduce immune activation; many of them are used to prevent organ rejection during and after transplants. These drugs, including methotrexate, Imuran, cyclosporine, infliximab (Remicade), eternacept (Enbrel), and adalimumab (Humira), are now commonly used to treat autoimmune diseases such as inflammatory bowel disease, psoriasis, and rheumatoid arthritis. However, they can cause dangerous side effects. They can also deactivate the immune system to the point of putting one at risk for contracting a serious infection. In fact, people who take these drugs are more prone to all infections, even those that normally wouldn't pose a problem.

The scientific research on how to control and enhance our immune function continues to grow rapidly. When the final pieces are in place, we'll gain greater control over our immune system, which will allow us to be free of infections, to prevent illness, and to stop and even reverse the aging process.

TAKE ACTION: ENHANCE

First and foremost, keep in mind that not everyone has to take every supplement. Read this as you might read a menu, looking over all the possibilities and selecting what is right for you—although at the end I will make recommendations for everyone.

One of the greatest challenges in enhancing the immune system is knowing which specific actions to take. If you tried to research, find, and ingest every supplement listed, you wouldn't have time for anything else. Nor can you take every test available—you'd probably become anemic from having so much blood drawn. But there must be some way of knowing exactly what you should do, and take, to enhance your immune function.

Fortunately, there is. The most reliable way to find out if you have a problem is by measuring your level of overall immune activation. At Canyon Ranch, we use the highly sensitive CRP test (hs-CRP), which is inexpensive and widely available. Our goal is to get that CRP level down as low as possible—ideally, less than 0.7 milligrams per liter. CRP levels as low as 0.2 milligrams per liter are not unheard of among the ultrahealthy.

Your CRP level, which your doctor can test for you, can be your guide to decide how aggressively you should pursue this Enhance step. If your CRP is 0.6 or below, you're doing a great job. Keep it up. If your CRP is between 0.6 and 3, you can take a low level of supplements: for example, a fish oil capsule, a multivitamin with some added vitamin D, and maybe a probiotic daily.

If your CRP is higher than 3, you're more at risk, so you'll need a more comprehensive approach. You might want to take a daily dose of 3,000 milligrams of fish oil, the full 1,000 units of vitamin D, and vitamins C, E, B6, and B12 in addition to ensuring an adequate intake of chromium, magnesium, selenium, zinc, and fiber.

If your CRP is drastically elevated (over 10, for example) as a result of a serious inflammatory condition, say rheumatoid arthritis or inflammatory bowel disease, you'd want to add a blend of herbal and phytonutrient supplements to help reduce the level of immune activation.

FIRST STEPS TO AN ENHANCED IMMUNE SYSTEM

1. **Get your baseline CRP level:** Take this step the next time you have a physical exam. Create a spreadsheet, or keep a journal, that keeps track of your CRP readings from all your physicals, as well as all your vitamins, medications, and supplements, so you can monitor how your levels change over time.

2. **Calculate your waist-to-hip ratio:** This is a good way to see if you are at risk for immune activation. You can do this in the privacy of your own home, with just a tape measure.

   Take two measurements. First, measure your waist circumference by placing the tape around your abdomen at your belly button. The tape should be tight enough to lightly indent the skin, but not so tight it presses into it.

   Next, take the same measurement at the hips. Divide the

first number by the second. For example, 32 inches divided by 39 inches yields a ratio of about 0.82. The target ratio is slightly different for men and women. For men it should be less than 0.9, and for women, less than 0.8.

People whose numbers come in over these levels are those who tend to put on weight around the middle; their bodies make more immune-activating cytokines such as leptin. It's especially important that these individuals get sufficient chromium, fiber, and fish oil.

(The waist-to-hip ratio is often quite low due to large hips; some people, particularly women, feel self-conscious about them. Yet large hips usually indicate a lower waist-to-hip ratio, and that in turn means lower CRP levels and less immune activation—so I am glad to see them.)

3. **Add a column to your spreadsheet:** Important measurements, including your weight and your waist and hip dimensions, should be part of your journal or spreadsheet. These measurements will be helpful in gauging how well your UltraLongevity program is working.

4. **Tally the daily total for each supplement you ingest:** Remember, these may be coming from different sources—for example, you will want to add up how much vitamin D is in your multivitamin, how much you take in other forms, and how much is in your diet. In addition to the resources mentioned on page 121, you can find comprehensive nutrient analysis at the USDA Nutrient Database, www.nal.usda.gov/fnic/foodcomp/search/.

5. **Keep track of important blood tests:** Include in your spreadsheet and/or journal any other blood tests that might be important, such as your white blood count or your sed rate. Your doctor can perform these for you.

GENERAL GUIDELINES

Following are some general guidelines to boosting the power of your immune system.

FOR EVERYONE

- Everyone should be taking a multivitamin.
- We should all be getting 20 grams of fiber for every 1,000 calories we eat per day.
- We should all hydrate often.
- Those of us living in temperate, northerly latitudes, or who don't get out in the direct sunshine daily, should take additional vitamin D.
- Those who don't consume small, oily fish more than twice a week should be adding fish oil supplements.

FOR SPECIAL SITUATIONS

- If your family has a strong history of Alzheimer's disease and your CRP level is not ideal, along with your multivitamin add vitamins C and E and a B-complex vitamin.
- If you have a digestive problem that causes diarrhea or frequent loose stools, of if you are diabetic, take extra zinc.
- If you tend to gain weight around your middle (per the waist-to-hip-ratio test), add chromium to your program.
- If your blood pressure is borderline or elevated, consider L-arginine, especially if you are a male with some erectile dysfunction.
- If you have digestive symptoms, irritable bowels, or inflammatory bowel disorders, or suffer from other inflammatory conditions such as asthma or arthritis, add a probiotic daily.
- If you're diabetic, add lipoic acid, L-carnitine, zinc, magnesium, and possibly arginine (especially if your blood pressure is borderline high).

- If you have constipation, asthma, or migraines, add magnesium.
- If you have chronic hepatitis or other liver problems, consider milk thistle (silymarin).
- If you take anti-inflammatory or pain medications such as acetaminophen on a regular basis, add NAC.

By taking these steps to improve your internal environment and enhance the function of your immune system, you will be able to reduce the level of immune activation in your body while helping to prevent illness and decelerate aging.

A DAY IN THE LIFE OF THE
ULTRALONGEVITY PROGRAM

WHAT'S IT LIKE to live the UltraLongevity program? Imagine this scenario:

You wake up in the morning from a long, restful slumber. You now understand that the deep sleep that occurs right before you awake is the most valuable—and because you've just gotten a solid dose of it, you're feeling great, basking in a splendid sense of rejuvenation, well prepared to face whatever your day has in store.

You now do a few breathing exercises before leaving the bed, taking in at least three good, deep breaths. And you recite a small meditation. For many, morning is one of the day's few quiet moments, so you take a little time to contemplate something calming. Or perhaps you meditate with a mantra, coordinating it with your breathing. A positive thought in the morning can set the tone for the rest of the day.

If you're waking up next to someone, you know this is a great time to help him or her start the day off right too. You say a nice word, give a hug, show your love.

Now you slowly stand up and try a couple of stretches. You reach over your head, then down as far as you can, and stretch, spreading your legs out a little, arching your back a bit. As you're doing this, you take in some nice, mindful breaths. You know this is also a good time for an affirmation (I recommend one for everyone). You make a positive commitment to yourself: to stay on track with a healthy lifestyle, to continue your exercises, and to make a difference in the world.

You may be responsible for waking up others. If so, you don't wake them up like a rooster or an alarm clock. Because you want them to get up on the right foot, you wake them up with a message of love rather than a shout.

It's been several hours since you've had anything to drink. Dehydrated, you down a good eight ounces of water and then head off to the bathroom, where you perform your morning's ablutions.

On days when you're not rushed, you do the dance of the treadmill, or the dance of a home aerobics class. You know this is a good time to get up, out, and moving. Exercise helps wake you and gets your pulse rate up too.

Once your morning dance is finished, you take some of your daily supplements, your probiotic, and your vitamin D. And you take your shower. When you do, you grab the opportunity to sing. What a great way to elevate your mood. Croon at the top of your lungs!

Now you have your breakfast; here you choose something from the eight-day meal plan. As you eat, you do so mindfully, chewing completely, and sitting down (rather than standing up or running out the door).

With your breakfast, you sip a beverage, such as a cup of tea or coffee (you limit your caffeine to mornings). Ideally, if you're eating with others, you let them know how much you care for them. If they're not with you at the moment, you take time to think about your positive feelings.

If you have animal companions, you spend some time showing your warm feelings for them. They'll return that love right back to you. They always do.

Now your activities start. Whether it's a day for rest, errands, or work, you place your pedometer in your pocket or bag. You try to walk as much as possible, whether that means accompanying the kids to school or hiking up the two flights to your office instead of taking the elevator.

The morning flies past; soon it's time for your midmorning snack—today it's a banana. And you continue your mindful breathing—you check to make sure it's relaxed, slow, and appropriately deep.

If you're at the office, because you want your work area to be pleasant, you bring in some flowers. You're also careful to keep your windows open whenever possible for some fresh air.

As lunchtime nears, you take more supplements; for example, fish oil—having it right before lunch means you won't experience any of that fishy aftertaste that can occur when your stomach is empty. If you're taking a multivitamin twice a day, you take your first one now, as well as your amino acids or herbs.

For lunch you munch on a turkey wrap, making sure that you're not hurried and that you chew your food completely.

After lunch you take a short walk. At some point you feel tired—it's not unusual for fatigue to set in after a meal. To combat this, drink plenty of clean, filtered water. You know it's important to hydrate after lunch: Your body needs the water to help digest and process the food you just ate. You also avoid sitting down, because if you do, your body will slow down and you may lose focus.

Back in your office, you close the door and do a few back stretches by putting your hands on your hips and arching your back as you look up at the ceiling. You try touching your toes—or at least you reach toward them. You also spread your legs shoulder-width apart and then twist your torso right and left; this helps align your spine.

Later in the afternoon you crave a snack; today you try a trail bar.

At the end of your workday you do some shopping for dinner.

You also stop by a nearby animal daycare center to watch the puppies play. And you continue walking, registering those steps on your pedometer.

Before dinner you take your second multivitamin, as well as your second probiotic of the day and more fish oil.

For supper you chose one of the recipes from the eight-day meal plan—tonight it's the Chicken Fajitas. You also make sure dinner looks nice. You light a candle and play music. Ideally, you're eating with a friend or partner; you enjoy this time together, and you appreciate how lucky you are to have somebody in your life. But if you're alone, you make the dinner special just for you.

After dinner you check your pedometer for the day's activity and see that you're only at eight thousand steps, so you go outside for a short walk to make up for the two thousand steps left for the day. This helps your digestion and prevents you from feeling tired.

When you come back, you make a few entries in your journal. What are you feeling? How is your health? What are your plans for tomorrow?

Each night you choose a different way to soothe your immune system. Tonight you take a hot bath. First, you have a cup of chamomile tea, just to make sure you're really relaxed. You're gearing down and preparing for sleep. Now you give yourself credit: you did well today. After your bath, a good way to reward yourself is by engaging in your dream mantra, creating that wonderful, cozy space that will see you off to sleep. You make sure that your room is dark and quiet . . . soon you drift off.

The next thing you're aware of is waking up and lingering in those last few moments of deep, relaxing morning sleep, which is where we started.

Some people tell me that they're too busy to take care of themselves. Yes, you are busy. We all are. That doesn't mean we can't be healthy too.

None of the UltraLongevity program suggestions require much time, and almost all of them can be worked into your regular schedule. You can still be highly productive in your daily life even as you take care of yourself. For example, despite doing everything mentioned above, you could also have attended three meetings, fought with the rude person in the store, written five memos, talked to ten people, taken fifteen phone calls, walked your dog, and helped your kids with homework.

Far too frequently people take a reactive approach to their health. They wait until something goes wrong. They wait until they have a heart attack. They wait until they have cancer. Then they try to take care of it. Often, by that time, it's too late.

The road to health is through action, not avoidance. If you follow these seven UltraLongevity steps, you will be personally responsible for improving your health and slowing the process of aging, and you will live as long, and as well, as possible.

PART III

THE ULTRALONGEVITY EIGHT-DAY MEAL PLAN

EIGHT DAYS TO
A HEALTHY DIET

TO LIVE A long and healthy life, you must know how to eat well. But that doesn't always translate into *what* to eat. In other words, you may already know to eat slowly, to chew your food completely, to spread your calories out over the day, and to enjoy company during a meal—but that still leaves the question of what specific foods to choose.

To help, here is an eight-day UltraLongevity meal plan that combines the science of UltraLongevity with the principles of healthy eating. The meals are healthful, nutritious, and delicious. Each plan provides for a daily calorie intake of about 1,650 calories, the recommended amount for the average physically active forty-five-year-old, 125-pound woman. Other people should vary the serving sizes to reach their own recommended calorie intake.

(To estimate your daily calorie requirements, use this very general but fairly reliable rule: multiply your weight by eleven. If you're a regular exerciser, add the number of calories you typically burn during exercise.)

These meals also provide about 32 grams of fiber per day, which, as you have learned, is vitally important to your health. What you will also learn is that by eating these fiber-rich meals, you will find yourself feeling full even though you've consumed fewer calories than you used to.

Caveat: this isn't fast food. Shopping, preparing, and cooking healthy meals requires time and energy, but there's a payoff: a healthier immune system and a longer life.

We certainly don't expect many people to follow every meal suggested, every day, although if you did you would be eating extremely well. These meals are offered as guidelines for what you can do if you are operating at peak efficiency in the kitchen.

For most readers: Know that these meal plans can be switched or swapped—if you find one dinner recipe you love, and your family and/or friends love it too, then you'll probably prepare it more often than not.

Also keep in mind that for many people, cooking one meal one night means eating leftovers for the next day or more. I know one family who always doubles the recipe and then snacks on it for days to follow.

Use common sense here. You don't want to cook up a week's worth of food in one night, but keep in mind that a little work done one day can provide relief from the kitchen the next.

Furthermore, many of these dishes can be made in advance and stored, so you can cook when you have time and freeze or store meals or snacks to eat later. You can also double or triple the recipe ingredients so you're sure to have plenty for later. Few people have the time and the wherewithal to cook at the same time every night for the same number of people. Cook when you can and enjoy it when you want to.

Here are some basic rules of thumb regarding our meal plans, and some guidelines to help you in your own menu planning and shopping.

- These meals have about 20 grams of dietary fiber for every 1,000 calories.

- The spices and other ingredients chosen help to enhance the immune system.

- The meals are generally about 55 percent carbohydrate, 25 percent fat, and 20 percent protein, and they are low in saturated (animal) fats.

- Calories from fat should be from sources such as olive oil, flax or other omega-3 oils (fish, e.g.), and nuts (monounsaturated fats), all of which help to enhance immune function.

- You should eat fish more than twice a week.

- Choose whole grains over refined grains—for instance, whole wheat instead of white flour, brown rice instead of white rice, whole ("steel-cut") oatmeal instead of refined oatmeal.

- Fiber grams should exceed sugar grams on any packaged foods.

- Avoid "trans" or "hydrogenated" fats at all costs.

- Look for natural or organic products that are unrefined or minimally refined.

- Be careful about processed food products.

- Shopping in natural foods stores or stores that have whole foods sections will provide you with the most options (e.g., Whole Foods, Trader Joe's, Wild Oats, and local co-ops). Many of these grocery stores also have cafés where good prepared meals can be bought and eaten.

- Nuts and natural nut butters are great food choices for substituting—one of my favorite sandwiches is almond butter and bananas on spelt.

• Breakfast cereals should contain more fiber than sugar grams and should be natural without preservatives. Choose, for example, Uncle Sam's cereal, Ezekiel's, or other similar brands.

• Beware of the many names of sweeteners—high fructose corn syrup, fruit juice concentrate, molasses, honey, cane juice, etc.

Feel free to invent your own meals according to these guidelines. Write down your own recipes so you can duplicate them if you like them. Be creative.

A few more points to remember:

• Snacks are permitted but not mandatory. Let your hunger be your guide. The same holds true for dessert. No law says a dessert must come with every dinner. In fact, several dinner plans don't include one, to help you avoid making dessert a habit.

• Drink ample amounts of fluids with meals. Water is the best choice; if you wish to add a little flavor, consider dropping in a wedge of fruit, such as lemon or lime. You can also enjoy tea, coffee, or bottled sparkling water (but watch your caffeine intake after lunch).

• When choosing juices, look for natural ones without added sugar (e.g., most cranberry juices are excessively sweetened). Juices can also be mixed with water or sparkling water to reduce sugar intake while improving your hydration.

• Eat slowly and chew completely. You've taken the time to prepare a wonderful meal. Savor it.

• Share your culinary creations with friends and family. It's easier to cook for more than one, and most of these recipes are designed for several servings. If your friends can't join you, refrigerate or freeze the extra servings for a future meal.

- Finally, if you've been through the rotation several times and are becoming bored, experiment. You've learned enough about healthy cooking to create your own dishes according to the principles of UltraLongevity.

Think about it. Not only do you get to savor the wonderful foods that are so wholesome and nourishing, you're keeping yourself young by doing so. Eat well, and live long! Bon appétit!

DAY 1

BREAKFAST

Egg White Omelet with Vegetables

Serve with ¼ cup of your favorite organic salsa and a slice of multigrain toast.

3 egg whites
½ teaspoon canola oil
¼ cup diced bell pepper
1 tablespoon diced green onion tops

½ cup sliced white mushrooms
¼ medium tomato, diced
1 tablespoon low-fat Monterey Jack cheese

1. In a small mixing bowl, whisk the egg whites just until they become frothy.
2. Lightly coat a small skillet with canola oil, and sauté vegetables over medium-high heat until tender.
3. Pour egg mixture over vegetables. As the eggs start to set, use a spatula to lift edge of eggs and allow uncooked portion to run under the cooked portion. This makes the omelet cook more evenly throughout. As soon as all the mixture has set, sprinkle cheese on vegetables, remove the pan from the heat, and fold omelet in half. Serve immediately.

NOTE: You can substitute any of your favorite vegetables.

Makes 1 serving, containing approximately:
130 calories • 9 gm carbohydrate • 5 gm fat • 8 mg cholesterol • 15 gm protein • 230 mg sodium • 2 gm fiber

Without cheese:
95 calories • 8 gm carbohydrate • 3 gm fat • 0 mg cholesterol • 11 gm protein • 145 mg sodium • 2 gm fiber

NUTRITIONAL NOTE: Whole Egg Omelet with Vegetables (3 eggs, no cheese) supplies approximately 260 calories, 17 gm fat, 639 mg cholesterol.

MIDMORNING SNACK

One-eighth cup (2 tablespoons) walnuts.

LUNCH

Tortilla Soup

4 *large Roma (plum) tomatoes,*
sliced
2 *medium onions, sliced*
½ *tablespoon olive oil*
½ *cup diced celery*
1 *teaspoon minced jalapeño pepper*
¼ *cup diced green chilies*
1 *teaspoon minced fresh garlic*
½ *teaspoon chili powder*
2½ *teaspoons ground cumin*
1 *teaspoon minced cilantro*

2 *tablespoons tomato paste*
¼ *teaspoon sugar*
1 *quart Vegetable Stock (see*
recipe below) or canned or frozen
vegetable stock
1 *teaspoon salt, optional*
6 *teaspoons nonfat sour cream*
6 *tablespoons shredded low-fat*
Monterey Jack cheese
1 *blue corn tortilla, julienned*
3 *tablespoons chopped cilantro*

1. Preheat oven to 350°F. Lightly coat a sheet pan with a small amount of canola oil.
2. Spread tomatoes and onions on sheet pan. Roast in oven 15 to 20 minutes, or until vegetables begin to turn brown on the edges.
3. Meanwhile, heat olive oil in a large saucepan over medium heat and add celery, jalapeño, and chilies. Reduce heat and simmer 2 to 3 minutes. Add garlic and cook another 2 minutes, or until garlic starts to turn golden brown.
4. Add spices and minced cilantro and cook 1 more minute. Add tomato paste and sugar and cook until tomato paste turns rust-colored, 3 to 4 minutes. A small amount of water may be added to prevent sticking. Add roasted tomatoes and onions and mix well.
5. Add Vegetable Stock and bring to a low boil. Cook 5 more minutes. Cool briefly. Add salt, if desired, and puree in blender or food processor until smooth. Strain if desired.

6. Garnish each serving with 1 teaspoon nonfat sour cream, 1 tablespoon cheese, 1 tablespoon tortilla strips, and ½ tablespoon chopped cilantro.

Makes 6 (¾-cup) servings, each containing approximately:
    115 calories • 20 gm carbohydrate • 3 gm fat • 4 mg cholesterol •
    5 gm protein • 359 mg sodium • 4 gm fiber

Vegetable Stock

2 medium leeks, washed and
  chopped
4 onions, chopped
6 carrots, peeled and chopped
1 small bunch celery, chopped

1 small bunch parsley, chopped
3 bay leaves
2 teaspoons dried leaf marjoram
½ teaspoon dried thyme
6 quarts cold water

1. Combine all ingredients in a large stockpot and bring to a boil. Reduce heat and simmer uncovered 1 hour, skimming off any foam that comes to the surface. Do not stir, and do not allow to boil again. Let stock cool slightly for easier handling.
2. Line a kitchen strainer or colander with a double thickness of cheese-cloth and set over a very large bowl or pot in the kitchen sink. Strain stock through cheesecloth, pouring slowly and steadily so as to not stir up sediments. Discard the dregs. Cool.
3. Refrigerate or store in the freezer in small portions.

Makes 16 (1-cup) servings, each containing approximately:
    10 calories • 3 gm carbohydrate • Trace fat • 0 mg
    cholesterol • Trace protein • 21 mg sodium • Trace fiber

NOTE: For sweeter stock add bell peppers, zucchini, and yellow squash. Do not add cabbage, lettuce, or eggplant, as they cause bitterness. Also, if you prefer, you can buy excellent vegetable stock in cans, or frozen, and substitute it for homemade.

Grilled Vegetable Wrap

1 medium red bell pepper
1 medium yellow bell pepper
1 small eggplant
2 large portobello mushrooms
4 fresh pineapple rings, ½-inch slices
1 tablespoon balsamic vinegar

1 tablespoon dried oregano
1 tablespoon dried basil
4 whole wheat tortillas, about
  9 inches in diameter
4 cups chopped romaine lettuce

1. Preheat grill.
2. Cut bell peppers into quarters and remove ends and seeds. Peel eggplant and slice lengthwise. Stem portobello mushrooms.
3. Grill vegetables and pineapple rings until tender. Remove and let cool.
4. Remove any loose skin from the peppers. Julienne vegetables and fruit and toss together in a medium-sized bowl with vinegar, oregano, and basil.
5. Place tortillas onto flat working surface. Spoon 1 cup vegetables and 1 cup romaine lettuce onto each tortilla. Roll tortillas, folding ends in, and cut in half on the diagonal.

Makes 4 servings, each containing approximately:
320 calories • 60 gm carbohydrate • 6 gm fat • 0 mg cholesterol • 10 gm protein • 453 mg sodium • 7 gm fiber

MIDAFTERNOON SNACK

One or two Canyon Ranch Trail Bars.

Canyon Ranch Trail Bars (Gluten-Free)

1 cup almond butter
1 cup brown rice syrup
¾ cup chopped almonds
1 cup dried cherries
1⅔ cup puffed millet

1⅔ cup puffed rice
¼ cup pumpkin seeds
¾ cup sunflower seeds
⅓ cup quinoa flakes (see note)

1. Lightly coat a 9 × 13-inch baking pan with canola oil.
2. In a large saucepan, heat almond butter with brown rice syrup over low heat until bubbles form. Quickly stir in remaining ingredients and mix well. Remove from heat.
3. When cool enough to handle, press into baking pan. Cool completely. Cut into 40 bars.

NOTE: Quinoa flakes can be found in natural food markets in the cooked cereal section. Compared with other grains, quinoa is a balanced source of protein and complex carbohydrates.

Makes 40 servings, each containing approximately:
130 calories • 15 gm carbohydrate • 7 gm fat • 0 mg cholesterol • 3 gm protein • 2 mg sodium • 1 gm fiber

DINNER

Asian Cabbage Rolls with Mongolian BBQ Sauce

½ cup julienned carrot
½ cup diced red bell pepper
½ cup julienned celery
½ cup sliced shiitake mushrooms
½ cup bean sprouts
1½ cups shelled edamame

1 tablespoon canola oil
1 tablespoon sesame oil
¾ cup Mongolian BBQ Sauce
  (see recipe below)
8 large napa cabbage leaves
2 cups cooked brown rice

1. In a large mixing bowl, combine carrot, red bell pepper, celery, mushrooms, bean sprouts, and edamame. Steam vegetables in a steamer or in a steamer basket over boiling water, covered, for 5 minutes.
2. Remove steamed vegetables and return to the mixing bowl. Add canola oil, sesame oil, and 3 tablespoons of the Mongolian BBQ Sauce and mix together.
3. Place napa cabbage leaves in a steamer or in a steamer basket over boiling water, cover, and steam 1 minute, or until soft.
4. Lay 1 steamed cabbage leaf on a flat surface and place ½ cup vegetable filling inside one edge. Roll tightly. Repeat with remaining cabbage leaves.
5. For each serving, place ½ cup brown rice in the center of a plate. Arrange 2 Asian Cabbage Rolls on either side of rice and serve 2 tablespoons Mongolian BBQ sauce in a small ramekin on the side.

Makes 4 servings, each containing approximately:
  305 calories • 39 gm carbohydrate • 12 gm fat • 0 mg
cholesterol • 13 gm protein • 632 mg sodium • 6 gm fiber

Mongolian BBQ Sauce

½ cup low-sodium tamari sauce
2 tablespoons sugar
¼ cup rice vinegar
1 tablespoon sesame oil
½ cup sake
⅓ cup water
⅓ cup catsup
Pinch dried coriander leaves

Pinch ground ginger
¼ teaspoon red chili flakes
¼ cup minced leeks
2 teaspoons minced fresh garlic
2 teaspoons minced fresh ginger
2 tablespoons water
2 tablespoons low-sodium tamari
  sauce

1. In a large saucepan, combine ½ cup tamari, sugar, rice vinegar, sesame oil, sake, and ⅓ cup water and bring to a boil. Add catsup, coriander leaves, ginger, and red chili flakes. Simmer for 10 minutes. Remove from heat.
2. In a small bowl, combine leeks, garlic, fresh ginger, 2 tablespoons water, and 2 tablespoons tamari sauce. Add to cooked mixture and stir until combined. Store covered in the refrigerator.

Makes 16 (2-tablespoon) servings, each containing approximately:
   35 calories • 4 gm carbohydrate • Trace fat • 0 mg cholesterol • Trace protein • 288 mg sodium • Trace fiber

Sole with Lemon Grass–Red Bell Pepper Salad

Lemon Grass–Red Bell Pepper Salad:
3 red bell peppers, roasted and thinly sliced
3 tablespoons minced lemon grass
1½ tablespoons sherry vinegar
¾ teaspoon salt
¼ teaspoon black pepper

Sole:
4 sole fillets, about 4 ounces each
¼ teaspoon salt
¼ teaspoon black pepper
1 tablespoon olive oil

1. In a medium bowl combine all ingredients for Lemon Grass–Red Bell Pepper Salad and mix well. Set aside.
2. Season fish with salt and pepper. Sauté in a large sauté pan in olive oil, about 3 to 5 minutes on each side, or until cooked through. Serve 1 fish fillet with ⅓ cup Lemon Grass–Red Bell Pepper Salad.

Makes 4 servings, each containing approximately:
   180 calories • 9 gm carbohydrate • 6 gm fat • 54 mg cholesterol • 23 gm protein • 461 mg sodium • 2 gm fiber

DESSERT

Cranberry Apple Betty

8 teaspoons Inn Maid granola
4 teaspoons apple juice
2 teaspoons canola oil

1½ cups chopped apple
1 cup cranberries
½ cup apple juice concentrate

1. Preheat oven to 350°F.
2. In a small bowl, mix together granola, apple juice, and canola oil until crumbly. Set aside.
3. Place ⅓ cup chopped apple and ¼ cup washed cranberries into each of 4 custard cups. Spoon 2 tablespoons apple juice concentrate over fruit in each custard cup. Divide granola mixture into 4 equal portions and distribute evenly over fruit.
4. Bake 20 minutes, or until apples are tender and top turns golden.

Makes 4 servings, each containing approximately:
140 calories • 29 gm carbohydrate • 3 gm fat • 0 mg cholesterol • 1 gm protein • 8 mg sodium • 2 gm fiber

DAY 2

BREAKFAST

Two Canyon Ranch Trail Bars (see page 241), plus one large grapefruit or orange.

As always, be sure to include a beverage of your choice: consider tea, juice, water, or coffee.

MIDMORNING SNACK

Lavash crackers with hummus.

LUNCH

Cream of Broccoli Soup

¼ cup chopped onion
¼ cup chopped shallots
1 teaspoon minced fresh garlic
1½ teaspoons olive oil
1½ tablespoons chopped pistachios
½ medium potato, peeled and diced
½ teaspoon curry powder

Pinch turmeric
2 cups Vegetable Stock (see page 240) or canned or frozen vegetable stock
2 cups chopped broccoli
½ teaspoon salt
Pinch white pepper

1. In a medium saucepan, sauté onions, shallots, and garlic in oil until translucent. Add pistachios, potatoes, curry powder, and turmeric and cook over low heat 5 minutes.
2. Deglaze with Vegetable Stock and bring to a boil. Add broccoli and simmer over medium heat 15 minutes. Cool slightly.
3. Transfer mixture to blender or food processor and puree until smooth. Add salt and pepper.

NOTE: To thicken with cornstarch (if necessary), combine equal amounts of cornstarch and water to make a thin paste. Add ½ teaspoon at a time to simmering soup to thicken.

Makes 4 (¾-cup) servings, each containing approximately:
100 calories • 13 gm carbohydrate • 4 gm fat • 0 mg cholesterol • 5 gm protein • 266 mg sodium • 3 gm fiber

Southwest Grilled Chicken Quesadillas with Avocado Salad

Avocado Salad:
½ cup diced avocado
⅓ cup diced tomato
1 tablespoon diced red onion
2 teaspoons chopped cilantro
2 teaspoons lime juice
¼ teaspoon salt
½ teaspoon minced jalapeño

Chicken Quesadillas:
1 pound skinless chicken breast halves, boned and defatted
1 yellow bell pepper, thinly sliced
1 red bell pepper, thinly sliced
½ red onion, thinly sliced
1 teaspoon canola oil
4 whole wheat tortillas, about 9 inches in diameter
1 cup shredded low-fat Monterey Jack cheese

1. Combine all ingredients for Avocado Salad in a small bowl. Mix well and refrigerate.
2. Preheat oven to 400°F. In a large sauté pan, sauté peppers and onions in canola oil over medium heat until tender, 1 to 2 minutes. Remove from pan and set aside.
3. Add chicken breasts to sauté pan and sear 1 to 2 minutes on each side, or until golden brown. Transfer to a baking pan and bake in oven 10 minutes. Slice into 1-inch slices.
4. Place tortillas on a flat surface and divide the chicken among them,

placing it on half of each tortilla. Top each with ½ cup sautéed vegetables and ¼ cup shredded cheese. Fold tortillas in half. Place quesadillas on hot grill pan or under broiler to warm. Cut each one into 4 wedges. Serve with ¼ cup Avocado Salad alongside.

Makes 4 servings, each containing approximately:
365 calories • 28 gm carbohydrate • 14 gm fat • 69 mg cholesterol • 31 gm protein • 590 mg sodium • 4 gm fiber

MIDAFTERNOON SNACK

A banana or a piece of your favorite fruit, along with water or your choice of beverage.

DINNER

Spinach Salad with Pecans

½ cup seedless red grapes, cut in half *⅓ cup Balsamic Dijon Dressing*
6 cups organic spinach, cleaned *(see recipe below)*
2 tablespoons chopped pecans

Combine all ingredients in a bowl and toss. Divide into 4 equal servings.

Makes 4 servings, each containing approximately:
95 calories • 10 gm carbohydrate • 5 gm fat • 0 mg cholesterol • 3 gm protein • 172 mg sodium • 3 gm fiber

Balsamic Dijon Dressing

2 tablespoons canola oil or olive oil *½ teaspoon minced fresh garlic*
6 tablespoons balsamic vinegar *1½ tablespoons low-sodium tamari*
1½ cups vegetable stock *sauce*
2 tablespoons chopped shallots *Pinch of black pepper*
2 tablespoons Dijon mustard *1 tablespoon rice vinegar*
1½ tablespoons white grape juice *1 tablespoon cornstarch*
1 teaspoon whole-grain mustard *1 tablespoon water*

1. Combine all ingredients except cornstarch and water in a medium saucepan or bowl. Mix well with a whisk.
2. Bring sauce to a boil. In a small bowl or cup, mix cornstarch with water to make a thin paste. Add to sauce mixture and cook, stirring, until slightly thickened, 2 to 3 minutes.
3. Remove from heat and cool. The dressing should not be too thick when hot, as it will thicken as it cools.
4. Allow to cool. Pour into a jar, cover tightly, and refrigerate up to 2 weeks.

Makes 10 (2-tablespoon) servings, each containing approximately:
35 calories • 3 gm carbohydrate • 2 gm fat • 0 mg cholesterol • Trace protein • 209 mg sodium • Trace fiber

Baked Sweet Potatoes

2 medium sweet potatoes or yams, about 12 ounces each

¼ teaspoon salt
Pinch black pepper

1. Preheat oven to 375°F.
2. Slice ends off sweet potatoes and cut in half lengthwise. Lightly season cut side with salt and pepper.
3. Double-wrap each sweet potato half in foil and place in oven. Bake 40 to 45 minutes, or until soft.

Makes 4 servings, each containing approximately:
170 calories • 40 gm carbohydrate • Trace fat • 0 mg cholesterol • 3 gm protein • 114 mg sodium • 5 gm fiber

Raspberry Cornish Hen

2 Cornish game hens
1 cup raspberries
2 cloves garlic, minced
1 tablespoon olive oil
1 teaspoon low-sodium tamari sauce

⅓ cup raspberry vinegar
⅓ cup plum vinegar
2 tablespoons sugar
1½ teaspoons chopped fresh mint
1 tablespoon cornstarch

1. Cut hens in half lengthwise and remove skin and wing bone. Place in a large shallow bowl.
2. In a blender container, puree the raspberries, garlic, olive oil, tamari

sauce, vinegars, and sugar until smooth. Add the fresh mint and mix by hand.

3. Pour ½ cup of marinade over hens and marinate in the refrigerator for at least 2 hours.
4. Strain remaining marinade though a fine-meshed chinoise or sieve. Combine marinade with cornstarch in a saucepan. Stir until cornstarch is completely dissolved. Bring mixture to a boil, reduce heat to a simmer, and cook 5 minutes to thicken. Remove from heat and set aside.
5. Preheat oven to 350°F. Lightly spray a baking pan with olive oil.
6. Place marinated hens in baking pan, reserving marinade. Cover hens and bake 30 to 40 minutes, until golden brown, or until juices run clear when thigh is pierced with a fork. Baste occasionally with reserved marinade, if desired.
7. Ladle 2 tablespoons of thickened sauce over each breast.

Makes 4 servings, each containing approximately:
150 calories • 16 gm carbohydrate • 5 gm fat • 45 mg
cholesterol • 10 gm protein • 73 mg sodium • 4 gm fiber

DESSERT

Banana Yogurt Smoothie

¾ cup fruit-flavored nonfat yogurt   ⅓ cup skim milk
1 teaspoon honey   Pinch ground cinnamon, optional
1 small banana

1. Combine all ingredients in a blender container and puree until smooth.
2. Serve in attractive glasses, garnished with a dusting of cinnamon, if desired.

Makes 2 servings, each containing approximately:
115 calories • 25 gm carbohydrate • Trace fat • Trace
cholesterol • 4 gm protein • 58 mg sodium • Trace fiber

DAY 3

Yogurt with Fruit and Nuts

1 cup plain organic nonfat yogurt   ½ cup blueberries
1 banana, sliced   ⅛ cup (2 tablespoons) walnut pieces

Combine yogurt, fruit, and nuts in a cereal bowl.

Makes 1 serving, containing approximately:
  371 calories • 86 gm carbohydrate • 11 gm fat • 5 mg
  cholesterol • 14 gm protein • 49 mg sodium • 7 gm fiber

MIDMORNING SNACK
Bake a batch of Whole Wheat Flaxseed Bread (recipe below) over the week-
end and you'll have it all week. Enjoy a slice with a tablespoon of fresh berry
preserves as an optional snack today.

Whole Wheat Flaxseed Bread

2¼ cups warm water (90° to 105°F)   1½ teaspoons salt
1 tablespoon brown sugar   ½ cup nonfat dry milk
2 tablespoons molasses   3 tablespoons vital wheat gluten
1 tablespoon active dry yeast   ½ cup high-gluten flour
1 cup ground flaxseed   3 cups whole wheat flour
2 tablespoons wheat bran   1 tablespoon canola oil

1. In a large bowl, combine water, brown sugar, molasses, yeast, ground
   flaxseed, and wheat bran. Let sit for 15 minutes, or until bubbly.

2. In another bowl, combine remaining ingredients except canola oil. Mix well. Add half of dry mixture to yeast mixture and stir to combine. Stir in oil. Add remaining flour mixture and mix on low speed with a dough hook or by hand until all ingredients are well combined, about 1 minute. Knead with dough hook or by hand for 5 minutes, or until dough is smooth and elastic and lightens in color.
3. Lightly coat two 8½ × 4½ × 2½-inch loaf pans with additional canola oil.
4. Place dough in a large bowl and cover with a towel. Let sit in a warm place until it doubles in size—about an hour. Punch dough down, divide in half, and shape into 2 loaves. Place in pans and let rise until doubled in size again—about another hour.
5. While loaves finish rising, preheat oven to 375°F.
6. Bake loaves at 375° for 15 minutes, reduce heat to 325°, and bake 30 minutes longer. Remove bread from pans immediately and let cool. Cut each loaf into 16 slices.

Makes 2 loaves (16 slices each), each slice containing approximately:
105 calories • 16 gm carbohydrate • 3 gm fat • 0 mg cholesterol • 6 gm protein • 122 mg sodium • 3 gm fiber

LUNCH

Bean and Vegetable Quesadillas

¾ cup dried black beans
¼ cup diced red onion
2 tablespoons diced leeks
1 tablespoon minced fresh garlic
2¼ cups Vegetable Stock (see page 240) or canned or frozen vegetable stock
½ cup salsa
¼ cup diced carrot
¼ cup diced red bell pepper
¼ cup canned diced green chilies, drained

2 tablespoons chopped cilantro
1 tablespoon minced parsley
1½ tablespoons fresh lemon juice
Pinch each of cayenne pepper, ground cumin, chili powder
4 whole wheat tortillas, about 9 inches in diameter
1 medium tomato, sliced into 8 slices
½ cup grated low-fat Monterey Jack cheese

1. In a large bowl soak beans overnight, covering with at least 3 inches of water. Drain and rinse.

2. Lightly coat a medium saucepan with olive oil. Sauté onions, leeks, and garlic until onions are translucent.
3. Add black beans and Vegetable Stock and bring to a boil. Lower heat, cover, and continue to cook at a simmer for 45 minutes, or until beans are tender.
4. Spray a small sauté pan lightly with olive oil. Sauté carrots, peppers, and green chilies until tender. Remove from heat and add cilantro, parsley, lemon juice, and seasonings. Mix well.
5. Transfer one-third of bean mixture to blender container and puree until smooth. Combine bean puree and beans with vegetable mixture.
6. Preheat oven to 350°F and lightly coat a baking sheet with canola oil.
7. Lay out 1 tortilla. Spoon ¾ cup mixture over half of tortilla. Lay 2 slices of tomato over filling and sprinkle 2 tablespoons cheese over tomato. Fold tortilla in half and lay on baking sheet. Repeat with remaining tortillas. Bake 6 to 8 minutes, or until hot. Serve each with 2 tablespoons salsa.

Makes 4 servings, each containing approximately:
320 calories • 48 gm carbohydrate • 9 gm fat • 8 mg cholesterol • 14 gm protein • 579 mg sodium • 10 gm fiber

MIDAFTERNOON SNACK

Dried fruit or veggie snacks from Just Tomatoes, Etc.! (available at justtomatoes .com—they have a wide variety of snacks, including organic options).

DINNER

Gingered Spiced Carrots

1½ cups finely diced Spanish or
  yellow onion
1 tablespoon olive oil
2 tablespoons minced fresh ginger
1 teaspoon ground cumin
4 tablespoons fructose

6 cups sliced carrot
2 cups Vegetable Stock (see page
  240) or canned or frozen vegetable
  stock
Pinch salt
2 tablespoons chopped fresh dill

1. In a large sauté pan, cook onions in olive oil over medium heat until onions turn a golden color.
2. Add remaining ingredients except for salt and dill. Simmer until carrots are tender.
3. Remove from heat and let cool 5 minutes. Stir in the salt and dill.

Makes 6 (½-cup) servings, each containing approximately:
110 calories • 26 mg carbohydrate • Trace fat • 0 mg cholesterol • 2 gm protein • 95 mg sodium • Trace fiber

Horseradish-Crusted Salmon with Cranberry Dill Catsup

Salmon:
⅓ cup all-purpose flour
1 teaspoon salt
1 whole egg, beaten
1 tablespoon white vinegar
1 cup finely grated fresh horseradish
Four 4-ounce salmon fillets
1 teaspoon olive oil

Cranberry Dill Catsup:
¾ cup fresh or frozen cranberries
½ cup apple cider
2 teaspoons minced shallots
Pinch salt
2 teaspoons sugar
2 teaspoons chopped fresh dill

1. In a shallow bowl, combine flour and salt and mix well. In a separate bowl, combine egg and vinegar and beat until combined. Spread horseradish in a medium shallow bowl. One by one, dip salmon fillets in flour mixture, then egg mixture, and then grated horseradish.
2. Heat olive oil in a sauté pan and sauté salmon over medium heat until cooked through and golden brown, 3 to 5 minutes on each side.
3. In a blender container, combine cranberries, apple cider, shallots,

salt, and sugar and puree until smooth. Stir in chopped dill. Serve 2 ounces Cranberry Dill Catsup with each salmon fillet.

Makes 4 servings, each containing approximately:
275 calories • 14 gm carbohydrate • 13 gm fat • 88 mg cholesterol • 24 gm protein • 463 mg sodium • 2 gm fiber

DAY 4

BREAKFAST

Multigrain French Toast

4 whole eggs
¾ cup egg whites
¼ teaspoon ground cinnamon
Pinch nutmeg
½ teaspoon vanilla extract

¼ cup 2 percent milk
9 large slices multigrain bread (about ¾ inch thick), cut diagonally
¾ cup maple syrup

1. Combine eggs, egg whites, cinnamon, nutmeg, vanilla, and milk in a blender container and mix until smooth. Transfer to a shallow pan.
2. Heat a large sauté pan over medium heat and lightly coat with canola oil. Dip both sides of bread slices into egg mixture and transfer to hot pan. (Do this in batches to avoid crowding pan.) Cook until golden brown on both sides. Serve 3 pieces with 2 tablespoons maple syrup.

Makes 6 (3-slice) servings, each containing approximately:
280 calories (may vary, depending on brand of bread used) • 51 gm carbohydrate • 3 gm fat • 72 mg cholesterol • 14 gm protein • 517 mg sodium • 4 gm fiber

MIDMORNING SNACK

A chocolate coconut Lärabar snack bar.

LUNCH

Spring Pea Soup

¾ cup diced onion
¾ cup diced leeks
½ cup chopped scallion
2 tablespoons olive oil
1 teaspoon minced fresh garlic
2½ cups shucked fresh English peas
  or frozen green peas, thawed

5 cups Vegetable Stock (see recipe,
  page 240) or canned or frozen
  vegetable stock (see note)
½ cup chopped chives
1 teaspoon dried mint
½ teaspoon salt
¼ teaspoon black pepper

1. In a large saucepan, sauté onions, leeks, and scallions in olive oil until onions are translucent. Add garlic and peas and sauté for 2 minutes. Add Vegetable Stock and bring to a boil. Reduce heat and simmer 30 minutes.
2. Add chives and mint and cook 5 minutes. Remove from heat and allow to cool slightly. Transfer to a blender container and puree until smooth. Add salt and pepper.

NOTE: If purchasing premade vegetable stock, choose a low-sodium brand.

Makes 8 (¾-cup) servings, each containing approximately:
  80 calories • 13 gm carbohydrate • 2 gm fat • 0 mg
  cholesterol • 4 gm protein • 161 mg sodium • 4 gm fiber

Cranberry Chicken Wrap

4 skinless chicken breast halves,
  boned and defatted
½ cup Cranberry Dill Catsup
  (see page 253)
½ cup diced celery
⅓ cup chopped pecans

¼ teaspoon sea salt
1¼ teaspoons sherry vinegar
Pinch black pepper
1½ teaspoons chopped cilantro
4 whole wheat tortillas, about
  9 inches in diameter

1. Grill or broil chicken breast 3 to 5 minutes per side. Dice chicken and set aside to cool.
2. Prepare Cranberry Dill Catsup.
3. Combine chicken, catsup, and next 6 ingredients (celery through cilantro) in a medium bowl and mix well.

4. Place tortillas onto a flat working surface. Spread ¾ cup of cranberry chicken salad in the center of each tortilla. Roll tortillas, folding ends in, and cut in half on the diagonal.

Makes 4 servings, each containing approximately:
345 calories • 32 gm carbohydrate • 14 gm fat • 44 mg cholesterol • 23 gm protein • 499 mg sodium • 4 gm fiber

MIDAFTERNOON SNACK
Washed organic snap peas (prepackaged).

DINNER

Steamed Vegetable Basket
Steam a basket of your favorite mixed vegetables. Think about peppers, squash, cabbage, broccoli, cauliflower, brussels sprouts, button mushrooms, eggplant, or any of your own favorites.

Mediterranean Pasta Sauce

4 cups julienned zucchini, about 1 pound
¾ teaspoon minced fresh garlic
1 tablespoon olive oil
2 cups chopped peeled tomato

2 tablespoons chopped fresh basil
4 teaspoons crumbled feta cheese
4 teaspoons sliced black olives
4 servings freshly cooked pasta

1. In a large sauté pan, sauté zucchini and garlic in oil over medium heat until zucchini is cooked through.
2. Add tomatoes and basil and simmer for approximately 10 minutes.
3. Save half the sauce for freezing or refrigerating for later use. Divide the remaining half into 4 portions and serve over freshly cooked pasta. Garnish each plate with 1 teaspoon of feta cheese and 1 teaspoon of black olives.

Makes 8 (½-cup) servings, each containing approximately:
70 calories • 7 gm carbohydrate • 4 gm fat • 25 mg cholesterol • 2 gm protein • 104 mg sodium • 4 gm fiber

Tilapia with Tomato Orange Salsa

Tomato Orange Salsa:
½ cup diced orange segments
1 cup diced tomato
¼ cup diced onion
¼ cup diced yellow bell pepper
1 tablespoon lime juice
¼ cup chopped fresh cilantro
½ teaspoon salt
½ teaspoon sugar

Avocado Puree:
½ cup mashed avocado
2 tablespoons chopped yellow bell pepper
¼ cup chopped red onion
2 tablespoons chopped tomato
2 tablespoons lime juice
¼ cup water
½ teaspoon chopped fresh garlic
½ teaspoon salt

Tilapia:
1 pound tilapia fillets, cut into 4 equal portions
¼ teaspoon salt
¼ teaspoon black pepper
1 tablespoon olive oil

1. In a medium bowl combine all ingredients for Tomato Orange Salsa and mix well.
2. In a blender container combine all ingredients for the avocado puree and puree.
3. Season fish with salt and pepper. Sauté in a large sauté pan in olive oil about 3 to 5 minutes on each side, or until cooked through. Serve 1 fish fillet with ⅓ cup Tomato Orange Salsa and ¼ cup avocado puree.

Makes 4 servings, each containing approximately:
    270 calories • 38 gm carbohydrate • 5 gm fat • 50 mg
    cholesterol • 20 gm protein • 385 mg sodium • 2 gm fiber

DAY 5

BREAKFAST

Top ½ cup Uncle Sam cereal with a cup of skim milk or soymilk. Add ½ cup blueberries.

MIDMORNING SNACK

One-eighth cup (2 tablespoons) unroasted almonds.

LUNCH

Fish 'n' Chips

1 teaspoon olive oil
1 pound potatoes, cut into wedges
½ cup whole wheat flour
6 tablespoons whole wheat bread
  crumbs
Pinch black pepper
1 egg white
Four 4-ounce sole or scrod fillets

Tartar Sauce:
⅔ cup soy mayonnaise
1 tablespoon sweet pickle relish
1 teaspoon fresh lemon juice
1 teaspoon minced fresh parsley
Pinch cayenne

1. Preheat oven to 450°F.
2. Lightly spray baking sheet with olive oil. Arrange potato wedges on one side, leaving enough room for fillets. Bake in preheated oven for 15 minutes, or until golden brown and just tender.
3. While potatoes are baking combine flour, bread crumbs, and pepper in shallow bowl.
4. In a small bowl beat egg white. Dip fillets in egg white then coat both sides of fish with flour mixture. Transfer to baking sheet with potatoes and continue to cook for 10 to 12 minutes, or until fillets are crisp.
5. Mix all ingredients for tartar sauce. Serve 1 tablespoon on each fish fillet. Refrigerate leftover sauce.

Makes 4 servings, each containing approximately:
280 calories • 30 gm carbohydrate • 6 gm fat • 46 mg cholesterol • 23 gm protein • 355 mg sodium • 2 gm fiber

MIDAFTERNOON SNACK

A glass (or two) of unsweetened fruit or vegetable juice.

DINNER

Waldorf Salad

1 cup chopped red apple
1 cup seedless red grapes
1 cup finely chopped celery
4 teaspoons chopped walnuts
¼ cup soy mayonnaise

1 tablespoon lemon juice
Pinch ground cinnamon
Pinch allspice
Pinch ground ginger

1. In a medium bowl, combine all ingredients and mix well.
2. Cover bowl and refrigerate until ready to serve.

Makes 6 (½ cup) servings, each containing approximately:
45 calories • 9 gm carbohydrate • 1 gm fat • Trace cholesterol • Trace protein • 145 mg sodium • 1 gm fiber

Mashed Sweet Potatoes

2 medium sweet potatoes, washed,
  peeled, and cut into 1-inch cubes
2 tablespoons frozen orange juice
  concentrate

½ teaspoon salt
¼ teaspoon black pepper
¼ teaspoon ground cinnamon
½ teaspoon vanilla extract

1. Place 6 cups water in a large saucepan and bring to a boil. Add potatoes and cook 10 to 15 minutes, or until potatoes are tender. Turn off heat. Drain water from pan and place back on burner for 30 more seconds to dry potatoes.
2. Add remaining ingredients and mash with a potato masher until all ingredients are mixed well. Potatoes will be slightly lumpy.

NOTE: For smoother sweet potatoes, beat with electric mixer on low until smooth.

Makes 6 servings, each containing approximately:
  110 calories • 25 gm carbohydrate • Trace fat • 0 mg
  cholesterol • 2 gm protein • 250 mg sodium • 4 gm fiber

Cardamom Grilled Chicken with Mango Lime Sauce

Spice Mix:
3 tablespoons ground cardamom
1 tablespoon black pepper
2 tablespoons salt
1 teaspoon ground cinnamon
¼ teaspoon cayenne

Six 4-ounce skinless chicken breasts, boned and defatted

Mango Lime Sauce:
1 mango, cleaned and diced
½ cup lime juice
2 tablespoons olive oil
1 tablespoon minced fresh ginger
½ cup nonfat plain yogurt
½ teaspoon salt
1 tablespoon diced jalapeño
1 tablespoon chopped cilantro

1. Prepare coals for grilling or preheat broiler.
2. In a small bowl, combine ingredients for spice mix.
3. Lightly pound chicken breasts to flatten. Dust each with about 1 teaspoon spice mix. Store remaining spice mix in an airtight container for future use.
4. Grill chicken 3 to 5 minutes on each side, or until juices run clear when pierced with a fork.
5. Combine all ingredients for sauce in a blender container except last 2 ingredients. Puree until smooth. Pour into a bowl, add jalapeño and cilantro, and gently stir.
7. Serve each chicken breast with ¼ cup sauce.

Makes 6 servings, each containing approximately:
220 calories • 9 gm carbohydrate • 8 gm fat • 72 mg cholesterol • 28 gm protein • 667 mg sodium • Trace fiber

DESSERT

Maple Orange Flan

Flan:
2 eggs
2½ egg whites
1¾ cups 1 percent milk
½ teaspoon vanilla extract

Maple Caramel Sauce:
2 tablespoons maple sugar
2 tablespoons water
¼ teaspoon orange juice
3½ tablespoons fructose
1½ teaspoons shaved orange zest
Pinch of salt

1. Preheat oven to 275°F. Spray the bottoms only of 6 custard cups with nonstick vegetable spray.
2. In a medium-sized mixing bowl, blend all ingredients for flan with a wire whisk.

3. Ladle ½ cup flan mixture into each custard cup. Place cups in a baking dish and add enough hot water to the baking dish to reach the level of the filling in the cups.
4. Bake in preheated oven 30 to 40 minutes, or until custard is firm. A knife inserted in the center will come out clean. Chill.
5. To make caramel sauce, combine sugar, water, and orange juice in a small saucepan. Bring to a quick boil to dissolve sugar. Reduce heat, add remaining ingredients, and simmer 2 minutes, until mixture becomes a golden color. Remove from heat and cool.
6. To serve, turn out the flans onto 6 plates. Drizzle 1 teaspoon of caramel sauce over the top of each.

Makes 6 servings, each containing approximately:
105 calories • 14 gm carbohydrate • 3 gm fat • 79 mg cholesterol • 6 gm protein • 130 mg sodium • Trace fiber

DAY 6

BREAKFAST

Two poached eggs, 2 Chicken Sausage patties (recipe below), and a cup of fruit salad.

Chicken Sausage

1 pound ground chicken breast	*1 tablespoon maple syrup*
⅓ cup peeled and finely diced red	*2 teaspoons dried sage*
apple	*1 teaspoon salt*
2 tablespoons olive oil	*½ teaspoon black pepper*
2 tablespoons finely diced onion	*½ teaspoon minced fresh garlic*

1. In a medium bowl, combine ground chicken with all other ingredients and mix well.
2. Form into 6 patties, using about ⅓ cup mixture for each.
3. Place patties in a large sauté pan. Sauté over medium heat until cooked through, about 3 to 5 minutes on each side, or until golden brown.

Makes 6 servings, each containing approximately:
    140 calories • 4 gm carbohydrate • 6 gm fat • 44 mg cholesterol • 18 gm protein • 440 mg sodium • Trace fiber

MIDMORNING SNACK

An apple or a piece of your favorite fruit.

LUNCH

Mulligatawny Soup

¾ cup peeled and diced potato
¾ cup peeled and diced carrot
½ cup diced celery
½ cup diced onion
3½ cups Chicken Stock (see recipe
 below)
1 teaspoon curry powder
Pinch salt
1 teaspoon black pepper

Pinch thyme
½ skinless chicken breast, boned and
 defatted, poached, and finely diced
½ cup finely diced apple
½ cup finely diced carrot
1 teaspoon minced lemon zest
⅓ cup cooked white rice
Pinch ground cinnamon

1. Combine potatoes, ¾ cup carrots, celery, onions, and Chicken Stock in a medium saucepan. Bring to a boil, then lower the heat and simmer until vegetables are soft, about 15 minutes.
2. Allow soup to cool briefly, then transfer to a blender container and puree until smooth. Return to saucepan.
3. Season soup with curry powder, salt, pepper, and thyme.
4. Add the diced chicken, apples, and carrots and the lemon zest. Simmer for 10 minutes. Add cooked rice and cook until heated through.
5. Ladle ¾ cup soup into each bowl and garnish with cinnamon.

Makes 6 (¾-cup) servings, each containing approximately:
 70 calories • 11 gm carbohydrate • 1 gm fat • 7 mg
 cholesterol • 5 gm protein • 231 mg sodium • 2 gm fiber

Chicken Stock
Buy chicken parts (wings, back, necks) from your butcher for stock or save chicken carcasses in the freezer until you're ready to make stock.

2 to 4 pounds chicken parts, except
 the liver
3 quarts cold water
1 to 2 carrots, scraped and chopped
1 to 2 celery ribs without leaves,
 chopped

1 large onion, cut into quarters
2 to 4 cloves garlic, cut into halves
1 bay leaf
12 whole peppercorns

1. Place chicken bones and parts in a shallow baking dish and roast in 350°F oven until golden brown, 35 to 45 minutes. Drain off excess fat and discard.
2. Transfer browned bones and parts to a large pot. Add 3 quarts cold water and bring slowly to a boil, skimming off any foam that rises to the top.
3. Add remaining ingredients and turn down heat to a simmer for 3 hours. Do not stir stock at any point.
4. Strain stock into a glass, ceramic, or metal container. Discard bones and vegetables. Place container in an ice bath until cooled completely, or refrigerate uncovered in metal, glass, or ceramic container until fat has hardened. Remove and discard fat.

Makes 8 (1-cup) servings, each containing approximately:
   10 calories • 3 gm carbohydrate • Trace fat • 1 mg
   cholesterol • Trace protein • 48 mg sodium • 0 gm fiber

Asian Duck Salad with Ginger Soy Dressing

Ginger Soy Dressing:
½ cup lime juice
1 tablespoon low-sodium tamari sauce
1¼ cups water
2 tablespoons honey
1 teaspoon minced fresh gingerroot
2 teaspoons minced fresh garlic
Pinch crushed red pepper flakes
1 tablespoon cornstarch

Asian Duck Salad:
½ pound boneless duck breast
1½ cups sliced shiitake mushrooms
4 cups shredded napa cabbage
1 cup snow peas
¼ cup chopped scallions
1 cup water chestnuts
½ cup enoki mushrooms
1 cup roasted red bell pepper, sliced
½ jalapeño pepper, seeded and diced
1 teaspoon crushed red pepper flakes

1. Combine all dressing ingredients except cornstarch in a small bowl and mix well. Set cornstarch aside.
2. Divide the dressing into 2 equal parts. Place duck breast in a shallow glass baking dish and pour the first portion of salad dressing over top. Cover and marinate in refrigerator for at least 4 hours, or preferably overnight. Refrigerate unused portion of dressing, covered.
3. When duck has finished marinating, place unused portion of dressing in a saucepan and bring to a boil. Thicken with the cornstarch. Remove from heat and divide into 2 equal parts. Set both aside to cool.
4. Remove duck from marinade and grill or broil until cooked through. Discard marinade. Cut cooked meat into ¼-inch-thick strips.
5. In a large bowl, combine shiitake mushrooms, cabbage, snow peas, scallions, water chestnuts, and enoki mushrooms. Pour one portion of the reserved cooked dressing over vegetables and toss until well mixed.
6. Divide the vegetable mixture among 4 bowls and top each serving with ¼ cup roasted bell peppers and 2 ounces of duck breast. Drizzle the remaining cooked Ginger Soy Dressing over the tops of the salads and sprinkle with red pepper flakes.

Makes 4 servings, each containing approximately:
215 calories • 29 gm carbohydrate • 6 gm fat • 41 mg cholesterol • 16 gm protein • 330 mg sodium • 6 gm fiber

MIDAFTERNOON SNACK

A banana or other fruit; don't forget water, tea, or juice.

DINNER

Steamed Vegetable Basket

Steam a basket of your favorite mixed vegetables, as you did for dinner on Day 4. Try some new ones this time, picking from peppers, squash, cabbage, broccoli, cauliflower, brussels sprouts, mushrooms, or any others you enjoy.

Grilled Salmon with Mongolian BBQ Sauce

½ cup Mongolian BBQ Sauce (see page 242)
Four 4-ounce salmon fillets

1. Combine BBQ sauce and salmon and marinate for 30 minutes to 2 hours.
2. Preheat grill or broiler.
3. Grill or broil salmon fillets 3 to 5 minutes on each side, or until fish is cooked through.

Makes 4 servings, each containing approximately:
    215 calories • 3 gm carbohydrate • 11 gm fat • 54 mg cholesterol • 19 gm protein • 389 mg sodium • Trace fiber

DESSERT

Apple Strudel

3 tablespoons cornstarch
4 tablespoons water
1½ pounds apples, peeled and sliced
3 tablespoons sugar
¾ teaspoon ground cinnamon
½ cup raisins

Pâte Brisée:
1 cup all-purpose flour
¼ teaspoon salt
3 tablespoons sugar
¼ cup cold butter
6 tablespoons ice water
1 egg white, beaten
1 teaspoon sugar

1. Preheat oven to 375°F. Lightly coat a baking sheet with a small amount of canola oil and set aside.
2. Mix cornstarch and 2 tablespoons of the water in a small bowl and set aside.

3. Lightly coat a sauté pan with a small amount of canola oil. Over medium heat, sauté apples with sugar, cinnamon, and remaining 2 tablespoons water. When apples are tender, stir in raisins. Add cornstarch mixture and cook until thickened. Remove from heat and cool.

4. Place flour in a medium bowl. Add salt and sugar and mix well. Add butter and cut into flour, using a pastry cutter, until butter is the size of small peas. Add water, 1 tablespoon at a time, mixing gently after each addition. Dough will begin to form a ball when enough water has been added. Gather dough with dry hands and form into ball. Let rest for 5 minutes. On a lightly floured surface, roll out pâte brisée into an 8 × 12-inch rectangle, with one of the long edges nearest you.

5. To assemble the strudel, spoon the apple mixture onto the pâte brisée. It's easiest to add the apple mixture along the edge of the dough nearest you. Then carefully roll the mixture inside the pâte brisée, forming a long, cylindrical strudel. Gently pinch the ends flat to keep the filling from spilling out while cooking.

6. Brush top of strudel with beaten egg white. Sprinkle with sugar and transfer to baking sheet.

7. Bake 35 to 40 minutes, or until top is lightly browned. Remove from oven and trim any extra pastry off the ends. Cut into servings.

Makes 10 servings, each containing approximately:
150 calories • 31 gm carbohydrate • 3 gm fat • 7 mg cholesterol • 2 gm protein • 101 mg sodium • 3 gm fiber

DAY 7

Two poached eggs and Blueberry Pancakes (recipe below).

Blueberry Pancakes

Pancakes:
1¼ cups all-purpose flour
½ cup whole wheat flour
2 tablespoons sugar
¾ teaspoon baking soda
1 tablespoon baking powder
¼ teaspoon ground cinnamon
1 whole egg
1 egg white
1¼ cups buttermilk
¾ cup water
1 tablespoon butter, melted
1¾ cups fresh or unsweetened frozen blueberries, thawed

Maple Glaze:
¾ cup maple syrup
4 tablespoons chopped walnuts
2 teaspoons orange zest
2 tablespoons orange juice

1. Combine flours, sugar, baking soda, baking powder, and cinnamon in a large mixing bowl.

270

2. In a separate bowl, lightly whisk egg and egg whites together. Add the buttermilk and water and stir until blended.
3. Add wet ingredients to flour mixture. Mix slightly and stir in melted butter. When mixed, gently stir the blueberries into the batter.
4. Spray a large skillet or griddle with nonstick vegetable coating. Heat surface, then pour 3 tablespoons of batter at a time onto griddle or skillet. Cook until the top of each pancake is covered with tiny bubbles and the bottom is brown. Turn and brown the other side.
5. To make maple glaze, combine all ingredients in a small saucepan. Cook for 2 minutes over low heat. Serve 2 tablespoons maple glaze with 3 pancakes.

Makes about 8 (3-pancake) servings, each containing approximately: 195 calories • 37 gm carbohydrate • 3 gm fat • 32 mg cholesterol • 5 gm protein • 177 mg sodium • 1 gm fiber

MIDMORNING SNACK

Plain organic yogurt with some berries or a little muesli.

LUNCH

Kamut Salad with Dried Cranberries

Kamut is a type of organic whole-grain wheat in the same family as durum wheat. It is used as an alternative to wheat in many dishes and has a sweet, nutty flavor.

1½ cups whole Kamut grain
½ cup chopped pecans
1 cup dried cranberries
2 oranges, peeled and sectioned
¼ cup orange juice
¾ cup diced red onion

½ cup diced celery
3 tablespoons red wine vinegar
Pinch salt
1 teaspoon low-sodium tamari sauce
½ teaspoon black pepper
1 tablespoon minced parsley

1. Place Kamut in a saucepan with 4 cups water. Bring to a boil. Reduce heat and simmer 45 minutes, or until soft. Drain off excess water, transfer to a large bowl, and let cool.

2. Place pecans on a sheet pan and bake at 350°F for 5 to 8 minutes. Remove from oven and add to Kamut along with all remaining ingredients. Stir until well combined.
3. Portion ½ cup onto a salad plate and serve.

Makes 12 (½-cup) servings, each containing approximately:
280 calories • 51 gm carbohydrate • 8 gm fat • 0 mg cholesterol • 6 gm protein • 99 mg sodium • 9 gm fiber

Open-Faced Turkey Reuben

4 slices Whole Wheat Risotto Bread
(see recipe below)
Eight 1-ounce slices cooked turkey
breast
4 tablespoons Thousand Island
Dressing (see recipe below)

4 tablespoons sauerkraut
Four 1-ounce slices reduced-fat
Swiss cheese

1. Turn on oven broiler and lightly coat a sheet pan with a small amount of vegetable oil.
2. Place a slice of Risotto Bread on sheet pan. Top with 2 slices of turkey breast, 1 tablespoon Thousand Island Dressing, 1 tablespoon sauerkraut, and 1 slice Swiss cheese. Repeat with remaining ingredients.
3. Broil in oven until cheese is melted and bubbly.

Makes 4 servings, each containing approximately:
335 calories • 28 gm carbohydrate • 12 gm fat • 63 mg cholesterol • 23 gm protein • 376 mg sodium • 4 gm fiber

Whole Wheat Risotto Bread

½ cup skim milk
2 tablespoons honey
¾ teaspoon salt
2 tablespoons olive oil
½ cup cooked brown arborio rice

1 teaspoon crushed mixed
peppercorns
1 tablespoon active dry yeast
½ cup warm water
3 cups whole wheat flour

1. In a large saucepan, heat milk to just below boiling, then add honey, salt, olive oil, cooked rice, and peppercorns. Cool to lukewarm.
2. In a small bowl, dissolve yeast in warm water and stir into the rice

mixture. Add half the flour and beat until smooth. Add the remaining flour to make dough easy to handle. Knead quickly and lightly to form a smooth and elastic ball.

3. Place the dough in a large bowl lightly coated with vegetable oil and cover with a damp towel. Set bowl in a warm place until dough doubles in size—about an hour.
4. Preheat oven to 400°F. Lightly coat an 8½ × 4½ × 2½-inch loaf pan with a small amount of vegetable oil.
5. Punch dough down, shape into a loaf, and fit into loaf pan. Cover the dough and allow it to rise until double in size again—another hour or so.
6. Bake in 400° oven for 5 minutes. Reduce heat to 350° and bake 20 minutes longer, or until golden brown. Remove from pan and cool on a wire rack. When loaf is cool, slice into 13 slices, not including the crusty ends.

NOTE: This recipe can also be prepared in your bread machine, following the manufacturer's directions.

Makes 13 servings, each containing approximately:
130 calories • 23 gm carbohydrate • 3 gm fat • 0 mg cholesterol • 4 gm protein • 74 mg sodium • 4 gm fiber

Thousand Island Dressing

¼ cup canola oil mayonnaise
⅔ cup nonfat sour cream
1 tablespoon minced shallots
¾ cup chili sauce
⅓ cup sweet pickle relish
Pinch salt
Pinch black pepper
⅓ cup skim milk

Combine all ingredients in a blender container and mix well.

Makes 16 (2-tablespoon) servings, each containing approximately:
55 calories • 6 gm carbohydrate • 3 gm fat • 4 gm cholesterol • 1 gm protein • 188 mg sodium • Trace fiber

MIDAFTERNOON SNACK

A few olives (just a few, they're salty!).

DINNER

Carrot and Raisin Salad

½ cup diced pineapple, canned in juice
1 tablespoon plain nonfat yogurt
1 tablespoon nonfat mayonnaise

2 cups grated carrots
¼ cup raisins
Lettuce leaves for serving
Mint sprigs for garnish

1. Drain pineapple, reserving 2 tablespoons juice. Set aside.
2. In a medium bowl, combine yogurt, mayonnaise, and reserved pineapple juice. Mix well. Stir in carrots, pineapple, and raisins. Mix well again.
3. Cover and chill thoroughly.
4. To serve, line 6 chilled salad plates with lettuce leaves, top with ⅓ cup of carrot mixture. Garnish with mint sprigs.

Makes 6 (⅓-cup) servings, each containing approximately:
55 calories • 14 gm carbohydrate • Trace fat • 0 mg cholesterol • 1 gm protein • 53 mg sodium • 1 gm fiber

Roasted Acorn Squash

2 large acorn squash, cleaned and cut into 4 wedges each
3 tablespoons maple syrup

1 teaspoon salt
1 teaspoon ground cinnamon

1. Preheat oven to 375°F.
2. Steam squash in a large saucepan with a steamer basket for 15 minutes.
3. Combine syrup, salt, and cinnamon in a small bowl. Remove squash from steamer and arrange skin side down on a baking sheet. Season each wedge with a teaspoon of maple syrup mixture. Bake in oven 15 minutes, or until syrup caramelizes.

Makes 8 servings, each containing approximately:
80 calories • 21 gm carbohydrate • Trace fat • 0 mg cholesterol • Trace protein • 159 mg sodium • 2 gm fiber

Olive Oil, Parmesan, and Black Pepper Pasta

8 ounces dry pasta
4 teaspoons extra virgin olive oil
½ cup grated Parmesan cheese

5 teaspoons coarsely ground black
pepper

1. Cook pasta according to directions on package.
2. In a large mixing bowl, combine pasta, oil, cheese, and black pepper, and toss until pasta is evenly coated.
3. Divide into 4 equal portions and serve immediately.

Makes 4 servings, each containing approximately:
485 calories • 85 gm carbohydrate • 8 gm fat • 5 mg
cholesterol • 17 gm protein • 80 mg sodium • 3 gm fiber

DESSERT

Pear Crisp

¼ cup rolled oats
½ cup whole wheat pastry flour
3 tablespoons brown sugar
2 tablespoons canola oil
¾ teaspoon ground cinnamon
¾ teaspoon nutmeg

¾ teaspoon apple juice
¾ teaspoon water
4¾ cups peeled, sliced, and diced
pears
5 tablespoons frozen apple juice
concentrate

1. Preheat oven to 425°F.
2. In a medium bowl, combine oats, flour, brown sugar, canola oil, cinnamon, nutmeg, apple juice, and water until crumbly. Set aside.
3. In a saucepan, over low heat, toss pears and apple juice concentrate. Cover pan and cook until pears are tender, about 5 minutes.
4. Spoon ½ cup pear mixture into each of eight 10-ounce custard cups, followed by 2 tablespoons oatmeal crumb topping. Bake in preheated oven for 20 minutes, or until top is golden brown. Serve warm.

Makes 8 (½-cup) servings, each containing approximately:
130 calories • 24 gm carbohydrate • 4 gm fat • 0 mg
cholesterol • 2 gm protein • 4 mg sodium • 3 gm fiber

DAY 8

BREAKFAST

A *large orange or grapefruit, and a Banana Berry Smoothie (see below).*

Banana Berry Smoothie

½ medium frozen banana
1 cup frozen berries
¾ cup almond milk
½ cup organic plain yogurt
1½ teaspoons finely ground pumpkin
  seeds or flaxseeds

1½ teaspoons raw wheat germ
1 tablespoon omega-3 oil
1 scoop protein powder, about
  2 tablespoons

Place all ingredients in a blender and mix until smooth and creamy. Chill or serve over ice.

Makes 5 (4-ounce) servings, each containing approximately:
  125 calories • 18 gm carbohydrate • 5 gm fat • 0 gm
  cholesterol • 5 gm protein • 36 mg sodium • 3 gm fiber

MIDMORNING SNACK

A *nice raw vegetable mix, maybe carrots, celery, and cauliflower. You can dip them in a little fat-free ranch dressing if you want some extra zip.*

LUNCH

California Turkey Wrap

6 cloves garlic, peeled
½ cup light cream cheese
¼ cup thinly sliced sun-dried
  tomatoes
2 tablespoons sherry vinegar
1 tablespoon sugar
1 pound portobello mushrooms,
  washed and destemmed

1 teaspoon olive oil
Four 4-ounce skinless turkey breast
  fillets, cut into 1-inch strips
2 lavash wraps, cut in half
2 cups green leaf lettuce, cleaned
  and torn into bite-sized pieces
½ cup diced roasted red bell pepper
1 medium tomato, cut into 4 slices

1. Preheat oven to 350°F. Lightly coat a small baking pan with canola oil. Place garlic cloves on pan and roast 15 to 20 minutes.
2. In a blender container, blend roasted garlic, cream cheese, and sun-dried tomatoes until combined. Set aside.
3. In a small bowl, combine vinegar and sugar. Place mushroom caps gill side up on a lightly oiled baking sheet. Brush vinegar mixture on mushrooms and roast for 15 minutes, or until soft. Allow to cool and cut into thin strips.
4. In a large sauté pan, heat olive oil over medium heat. Sauté turkey until golden brown and cooked through, 3 to 5 minutes.
5. To assemble each wrap, place ½ slice lavash bread on a flat surface. Spread one-quarter of cream cheese mixture on lavash to all corners. Top with ½ cup mixed greens, a portion of turkey strips, 2 tablespoons roasted red pepper, ⅓ cup portobello mushroom, and 1 slice tomato. Tuck one end in and roll into a wrap sandwich.

Makes 4 servings, each containing approximately:
  320 calories • 23 gm carbohydrate • 6 gm fat • 110 mg cholesterol • 41 gm protein • 278 mg sodium • 4 gm fiber

MIDAFTERNOON SNACK

One or two Canyon Ranch Trail Bars (see page 241).

DINNER

Mixed Green Salad with Sesame Ginger Dressing

Oven-Baked Croutons:
2 teaspoons water
1 teaspoon ground cumin
1 teaspoon chili powder
1 teaspoon garlic granules
1 teaspoon dried oregano
2 slices whole wheat or multigrain bread

1 pound mixed greens
1 cup yellow teardrop tomatoes
½ cup Sesame Ginger Dressing (see recipe below)
4 teaspoons roasted pine nuts

1. Preheat oven to 400°F. Lightly spray a sheet pan with olive oil.
2. In a small bowl, combine water with spices. Using a pastry brush, lightly coat one side of bread slices with spice mix. Cut bread into 1-inch pieces and spread on sheet pan.
3. Bake in oven 10 to 15 minutes, or until bread cubes are crisp and brown.
4. Combine greens and tomatoes in a large bowl. Divide into 4 equal portions and place on salad plates. Drizzle each salad with 2 tablespoons dressing and top with ¼ cup croutons and 1 teaspoon pine nuts.

Makes 4 servings, each containing approximately:
110 calories • 16 gm carbohydrate • 4 gm fat • 0 mg cholesterol • 4 gm protein • 196 mg sodium • 4 gm fiber

Sesame Ginger Dressing

4 cloves garlic
1 cup apple juice
1 cup rice vinegar
3 tablespoons sesame oil

1 teaspoon salt
1 teaspoon black pepper
1 tablespoon fresh ginger juice
  (see note)

1. Preheat oven to 350°F. Place garlic on sheet pan and roast in oven 10 to 15 minutes, or until golden brown. Cool and mince.
2. In a medium bowl, combine apple juice, vinegar, sesame oil, salt, black pepper, ginger juice, and roasted garlic. Mix well.

NOTE: For fresh ginger juice, grate fresh gingerroot, including peel, and squeeze out juice using a dampened muslin cloth or cheesecloth. Discard ginger solids.

Makes 16 (2-tablespoon) servings, each containing approximately:
40 calories • 4 gm carbohydrate • 2 gm fat • 0 mg
cholesterol • Trace protein • 297 mg sodium • Trace fiber

Chicken Fajitas

Marinade:
2 tablespoons low-sodium soy sauce
¼ teaspoon minced gingerroot
¼ teaspoon minced fresh garlic
2 tablespoons olive oil
⅓ cup finely chopped cilantro
Pinch chili powder
3 tablespoons beer, optional
½ teaspoon Tabasco sauce
½ orange, thinly sliced
½ lemon, thinly sliced
½ lime, thinly sliced
1 tablespoon minced parsley

4 skinned chicken breast halves, boned and defatted (about 1 pound)
1 cup sliced assorted bell peppers
4 whole wheat tortillas, about 9 inches in diameter
½ cup salsa
½ cup Guacamole (see recipe below)
½ cup light sour cream

1. Combine marinade ingredients in a shallow baking dish and mix well.
2. Place chicken breasts in marinade, turning to coat evenly. Cover and refrigerate for at least 2 hours, or as long as overnight.
3. Spray a medium sauté pan with nonstick vegetable coating. Sauté bell peppers over medium heat until tender.
4. Prepare hot coals for grilling or preheat broiler.
5. Lift breasts from marinade and grill or broil 3 to 4 minutes per side. Cut chicken into strips and divide into 4 portions. Serve each

portion with a whole wheat tortilla and 2 tablespoons each of salsa, Guacamole, and sour cream.

Makes 4 servings, each containing approximately:
  415 calories • 43 gm carbohydrate • 12 gm fat • 72 mg cholesterol • 35 gm protein • 618 mg sodium • 6 gm fiber

Guacamole

½ *cup julienned spinach*
⅓ *cup frozen peas*
1 ounce light silken tofu
1½ tablespoons lemon juice
Pinch salt
Pinch ground cumin
Pinch cayenne
Pinch chili powder
Dash Tabasco sauce

6 tablespoons peeled and mashed
  avocado
3 tablespoons peeled and minced
  tomato
2 tablespoons salsa
3 tablespoons minced white onion
1 tablespoon chopped cilantro
2 teaspoons chopped scallion

1. Steam spinach until wilted. Remove from heat and squeeze out excess water.
2. Briefly steam peas and rinse under cold water to retain green color.
3. In a large bowl, combine spinach, peas, tofu, lemon juice, seasonings, and avocado and stir until well mixed.
4. Fold in remaining ingredients and mix well.

Makes 8 (2-tablespoon) servings, each containing approximately:
  30 calories • 2 gm carbohydrate • 2 gm fat • 0 mg cholesterol • 1 gm protein • 127 mg sodium • 1 gm fiber

DESSERT

One cup fruit salad, your choice of seasonal local fruits, when available.

VEGETARIAN
SUBSTITUTIONS

FOR THOSE OF you who are vegetarians, here are a few options to substitute for dinner meals.

Cantonese Tempeh Stir-Fry

1 teaspoon finely chopped serrano
  chili (approximately 1 chili)
1 teaspoon sesame oil
3 tablespoons low-sodium soy sauce
2 tablespoons brown sugar
2 tablespoons sherry wine
¼ cup light catsup
½ teaspoon ground ginger
¾ cup Vegetable Stock (see page
  240) or canned or frozen vegetable
  stock
1 cup tempeh, cut into 1-inch pieces
  (about 8 ounces)

¾ cup cut-up onion (about ½ large
  onion, cut into thick slices and
  quartered)
1 tablespoon olive oil
2 teaspoons minced fresh garlic
4 cups broccoli florets
2¼ cups cut-up sweet bell peppers
  (approximately 3 peppers, red and
  yellow, cut into 1-inch squares)
½ cup scallions sliced in 2-inch
  pieces
2 tablespoons roasted peanuts
1⅓ cups cooked rice

1. In a large saucepan, sauté chili in sesame oil over medium heat, about
   1 minute.
2. Add soy sauce, brown sugar, sherry wine, catsup, ginger, and Vegetable Stock. Reduce sauce by one-third. Set aside.
3. In a hot wok (or sauté pan), sauté tempeh and onions in olive oil
   until golden. Add garlic and cook 1 minute. Add broccoli and bell
   pepper. Stir-fry 1 minute. Add scallions and peanuts and stir-fry

1 more minute. Toss with sauce. Continue to stir-fry until vegetables are tender. Do not overcook. Serve ⅓ cup cooked rice with each portion.

Makes 4 servings, each containing approximately:
351 calories • 50 gm carbohydrate • 10 gm fat • 0 gm cholesterol • 17 gm protein • 534 mg sodium • 9 gm fiber

Curried Tofu Salad in Pita

8 ounces extra firm tofu, diced
2 tablespoons soy mayonnaise
2 tablespoons nonfat plain yogurt
⅓ cup peeled and diced red apple
¼ cup seedless red grapes, chopped
2 teaspoons apple juice
3 tablespoons diced red onion
1 tablespoon chopped fresh parsley

1 teaspoon curry powder
¼ teaspoon salt
Pinch black pepper
2 whole wheat pita rounds, cut in
   half crosswise
4 lettuce leaves
4 slices tomato

1. Combine tofu, mayonnaise, yogurt, apple, grapes, apple juice, red onion, parsley, curry powder, salt, and pepper in a large bowl. Mix well.
2. Open cut edge of each pita half. Fill pocket with ½ cup tofu salad, 1 lettuce leaf, and 1 slice tomato.

Makes 4 pita sandwiches, each containing approximately:
235 calories • 20 gm carbohydrate • 14 gm fat • 6 mg cholesterol • 12 gm protein • 137 mg sodium • 6 gm fiber

Grilled Vegetable Strudel with Tomato Olive Sauce

Vegetables:
1 red bell pepper, seeded and quartered
1 yellow pepper, seeded and quartered
2 tomatoes, seeded and quartered
1 yellow squash, cut on the bias into ¼-inch slices
1 zucchini, cut on the bias into ¼-inch slices
1 eggplant, peeled and cut into strips
2 chopped artichoke hearts, marinated or fresh

Marinade:
2 tablespoons chopped chives
2 tablespoons balsamic vinegar
1 tablespoon olive oil
Pinch salt
Pinch pepper
2 tablespoons finely chopped fresh basil

6 sheets phyllo pastry
Tomato Olive Sauce (see recipe below)

1. Grill vegetables until tender. Remove from grill, dice, and place on a large plate.
2. Combine marinade ingredients and sprinkle over vegetables. Allow to marinate overnight.
3. Preheat oven to 375°F.
4. Layer the 6 sheets of phyllo on work surface, spraying each layer with nonstick vegetable coating before adding the next sheet. Arrange vegetables lengthwise along one long edge of phyllo sheets, leaving about $1\frac{1}{2}$ inches on each end. Fold the ends in, overlapping the vegetables to enclose ends of the filling. Roll the phyllo and filling over to form a strudel roll. Transfer to a baking sheet, seam down, and spray the strudel roll lightly with nonstick spray. Score with knife to form 6 slices.
5. Bake 25 minutes, or until golden brown. While strudel is baking, make the Tomato Olive Sauce.
6. Remove strudel from oven and allow it to stand for 5 minutes before slicing into 6 equal portions. Spread 4 tablespoons sauce on the bottom of each serving plate and arrange strudel portion on top of sauce.

Makes 6 servings, each containing approximately:
145 calories • 33 gm carbohydrate • 1 gm fat • 0 mg cholesterol • 6 gm protein • 330 mg sodium • 2 gm fiber

Tomato Olive Sauce

4 Roma (plum) tomatoes, quartered and seeded
1 small red onion, sliced in ⅛-inch rounds
1 teaspoon olive oil
1 clove garlic, minced
¼ cup Vegetable Stock (see recipe on page 240) or canned or frozen vegetable stock
1 tablespoon chopped Kalamata olives
1 teaspoon balsamic vinegar
Pinch salt
Pinch black pepper
1 tablespoon chopped fresh basil

1. Grill tomatoes and onions until tender. Place in a blender container and puree. Strain into a small saucepan and let simmer over low heat 10 to 15 minutes.
2. Heat olive oil in a small sauté pan. Sauté garlic until soft. Add tomato sauce, remaining ingredients, and cook until heated through.

Makes 6 (4-tablespoon) servings, each containing approximately:
10 calories • 2 gm carbohydrate • Trace fat • 0 mg cholesterol • Trace protein • 80 mg sodium • Trace fiber

Vegetarian Bean Chili

½ cup dried garbanzo beans
½ cup dried navy beans
½ cup dried black beans
½ cup dried adzuki beans
Pinch epazote (see note)
1 teaspoon minced fresh garlic
½ cup diced onion
½ cup diced red bell pepper
½ cup diced yellow bell pepper
2 shallots, diced
1 tablespoon olive oil
¾ teaspoon dried basil
Pinch ground cumin
1½ teaspoons chili powder

Pinch chipotle pepper powder
¼ teaspoon herbes de Provence
¼ teaspoon dried oregano
Pinch black pepper
2½ cups canned diced tomatoes
3 tablespoons tomato puree
1¾ cups tomato sauce
2 cups Vegetable Stock (see page 240)
    or canned or frozen vegetable stock
4 teaspoons minced green chili
2 tablespoons chopped cilantro
1 tablespoon chopped parsley
2 teaspoons molasses
½ teaspoon salt

1. Soak beans in abundant water overnight. Drain. Place in a large saucepan and add fresh water to cover by 2 inches. Bring to a boil and add epazote. Reduce heat to a simmer, cover, and cook for 1½ hours, or until beans are tender.
2. In another large saucepan, sauté garlic, onions, peppers, and shallots in olive oil until tender. Add dry spices and sauté briefly. Add tomato products and Vegetable Stock and bring to a simmer.
3. Add cooked, drained beans and return to a simmer. Add green chili and cook for 45 minutes.
4. Add cilantro, parsley, and molasses and cook for 5 minutes. Season with salt.

NOTE: Epazote, an herb from Mexico, is often used when cooking beans.

It is said to have an antiflatulent effect. You can find it in the Mexican food spice section of your whole foods grocery store.

Makes 10 (1-cup) servings, each containing approximately:
  175 calories • 32 gm carbohydrate • 2 gm fat • 0 mg
  cholesterol • 9 gm protein • 189 mg sodium • 7 gm fiber

Tempeh Fajitas

Marinade:
2 tablespoons low-sodium soy sauce
¼ teaspoon minced gingerroot
¼ teaspoon minced fresh garlic
2 tablespoons olive oil
Pinch chili powder
⅓ cup finely chopped cilantro
3 tablespoons nonalcoholic beer, optional
½ teaspoon Tabasco sauce
½ orange, thinly sliced
½ lemon, thinly sliced
½ lime, thinly sliced
1 tablespoon minced parsley

8 ounces tempeh, cut into lengthwise strips
1 bell pepper, cut into ½-inch slices
4 whole wheat tortillas, about 9 inches in diameter
½ cup salsa
1 cup Guacamole (see page 280)

1. Combine marinade ingredients in a shallow baking dish and mix well.
2. Place tempeh in dish with marinade, turning to coat evenly. Cover and refrigerate for at least 1 hour, or as long as overnight.
3. Lightly coat a medium sauté pan with a small amount of vegetable oil. Sauté bell peppers and tempeh over medium heat until tender.
4. Divide into 4 portions and serve each with a whole wheat tortilla, 2 tablespoons salsa, and ¼ cup Guacamole.

Makes 4 servings, each containing approximately:
  360 calories • 48 gm carbohydrate • 13 gm fat • 0 mg
  cholesterol • 16 gm protein • 598 mg sodium • 9 gm fiber

ACKNOWLEDGMENTS

THANKS TO THE many people who provided help, love, and support, writing this book has been a true labor of love.

I'd like to mention a few of these people: first off, my wonderful patients. Striving for optimal health, they have helped erase my misconceptions and have taught me what is possible. There's a reason they call it the "practice" of medicine, and I am grateful for the opportunity to learn from my patients.

I am also grateful for the support of my family, without whom this book would not have been possible: Siobhan, my wife, best friend, and confidante, and a brilliant physician; and the other sources of constant learning—my terrific, incomparable children, Timothy, Matthew, and Brenna.

I'd like to also thank my parents, Charles and Bess Liponis, who remain the ultimate role models after fifty-five years of joyful marriage.

My second family starts with Mel and Enid Zuckerman, the founders of Canyon Ranch. Their vision, integrity, and support are responsible for this information's getting to you, and I don't have words to express my gratitude. I'd also like to thank Jerrold Cohen, CEO of Canyon Ranch, who for fifteen years has been one of my biggest supporters as well as a dear friend.

Life is a continuous classroom, and I've been fortunate to have so many great teachers. These include the physicians on staff at

Acknowledgments

Canyon Ranch, including Drs. Cynthia Geyer, Stephen Brewer, Phil Eichling, Karen Koffler, Nina Molin, Stephanie Beling, Andy Plager, Todd Lepine, Jyotsna Sahni, Rich Gerhauser, and Bruce and Molly Roberts. Thanks also to the top nutritionists at Canyon Ranch, Lisa Powell and Lori Reamer, and to Dr. Mark Hyman.

Of course, many thanks go to my superb agent, Richard Pine, for his constant support and encouragement, and to my extraordinarily talented editor, Tracy Behar, at Little, Brown.

Finally, I'd like to thank Gene Stone for his tireless and superb work on this book. Gene's collaboration has been invaluable, and his friendship has been cherished.

INDEX

abdominal breathing, 88
acceptance, and emotional health, 163–164
acetyl-L-carnitine, 210
acidophilus (*Lactobacillus acidophilus*), 114, 217
adalimumab (Humira), 220
adiponectin, 100
advocacy, 176–177
aerobics, 155–156, 157
aging, 23–27, 28, 50, 54–55, 225
  diet and, 99, 106–107
  emotions and, 162
  exercise and, 142
  exposure to chemicals and, 192
  sleep and, 133
  spurts, 58–59
  supplements and, 199
  symbiotic/desirable bacteria and, 74
air pollution, 8–9, 184–187
alcohol, 125–126, 133, 139
allergens, 192–196
allergies, 31, 39
  air pollution and, 185, 187
  antibiotics and, 10–11, 216
  cockroaches and, 194
  dust mites and, 195
  eosinophil cells and, 44
  food, 104–105, 106
  hygiene hypothesis and, 77
  molds and, 193, 194
  See also allergens
alpha-lipoic acid. *See* lipoic acid
ALTs (associated lymphoid tissues), 45
Alzheimer's disease, 57, 77, 224
  elevated hs-CRP and, 52
  infections and, 64

music and, 150
  vitamin B12 and, 205
American Heart Journal, 8
American Journal of Cardiology, 9–10, 63
American Journal of Medicine, 8, 15, 201
*American Journal of Respiratory and Critical
  Care Medicine*, 185
amino acids, 109, 112, 208, 209–210
amyloid, 57
anaerobic exercise, 159
anger/hostility, 15, 69–70
  acceptance and, 163
  heart disease and, 162
  heart rate variability (HRV) and, 93
angiogenesis, 65–66
anti-angiogenesis therapy, 67
antibiotics, 10–11, 74–75, 125, 216–217, 218
antibodies, 38, 39, 40–41, 57, 73, 105, 131
  aging and, 54–55
  antinuclear, 191
  B cells and, 46
  coronary artery disease and, 63
  genes and, 68
  infections and, 54
  molds and, 193
antigens, 106
anxiety
  acceptance and, 163
  aromatherapy and, 183
  exercise and, 145
  healing-touch therapy and, 181
  heart rate variability (HRV) and, 93
  immune system activation and, 70
  insomnia and, 132
  meditation and, 152

Index

anxiety *(cont.)*
  music and, 149–150
  UltraLongevity quiz and, 16
apnea, 94, 183
  See also sleep apnea
aquariums, 198
Archives of Internal Medicine, 12
aromatherapeutic oils, 137–138
aromatherapy, 183, 197
arthritis
  infections and, 216
  leptin and, 101
  molds and, 193
  probiotics and, 224
  rhythmic movement and, 155
  vitamin D deficiency and, 202
  Whipple's disease and, 215
  See also rheumatoid arthritis
Art of Happiness: A Handbook for Living, The
    (Dalai Lama), 173
asbestos, 191
Aspergillus, 192
aspirin, 220
asthma, 39, 73, 125
  air pollution and, 185, 187
  antibiotics and, 11, 75, 216
  breathing and, 89, 91, 94
  caution about L-arginine and, 210
  cockroaches and, 194
  dust mites and, 195
  eosinophil cells and, 44
  magnesium and, 207–208, 225
  probiotics and, 224
  timing and, 148
atherogenesis, 144
atherosclerosis, 56
Atherosclerosis, 143
autoimmune diseases
  aging and, 23
  curcuminoids and, 218
  cytokines and, 47
  diseases caused by immune system, 5
  food allergies and, 105
  home water filter systems and, 191
  hygiene hypothesis and, 77
  infections and, 64, 65
  lipoic acid and, 211
  love and, 164
  lycopene and, 219
  medications and, 220–221
  mercury exposure in animals and, 192
  molds and, 193
  polyphenols and, 219

selenium and, 206
support groups and, 176
symbiotic/desirable bacteria and, 74
vitamin D deficiency and, 202
Aviation, Space, and Environmental Medicine, 184
Ayurveda, 134

back injuries, 152
bacteria, 28, 74–75
Baker, Dan, 173
ballroom dancing, 156
Bartonella henselae, 216
basophils, 44
B cells, 37, 38–41, 104
  antibodies and, 46, 54
  GALT (gut-associated lymphoid tissues)
    and, 45
  infections and, 54
  lymph nodes and, 37
bifidobacteria, 114, 212, 217
biking, 156, 159
biofeedback, 93
Biological Psychiatry, 70
birth, time of year of, 18
birth weight, 10, 18, 179
Blastomyces, 192
blepharitis, 215
blood pressure, 51, 52, 57, 59, 60, 71, 77, 101, 224
  built-in rhythms and, 148
  hostility and, 69, 162
  L-arginine and, 210
  magnesium and, 208
  plaque and, 56
  white-coat high blood pressure, 86
bone marrow, 33–34, 38
brain, 16, 57, 64, 146–147, 150
  breathing and, 92
  emotions and, 70–71
  endorphins and, 184
  lipoic acid and, 211
  sleep and, 127, 131
  Whipple's disease and, 215
Brain, 145
Brain, Behavior, and Immunity, 132
breathing, 60, 82, 84–98, 226, 228
  health and, 91–93
  improving mechanics of, 96–98
  love and, 175
  natural killer cells and, 43
  phases of, 89–91, 95
  rhythmic movement and, 147, 150
  sleep and, 136
  taking action for, 94–98

Index

types of, 86–88
why we breathe, 85, 88–89
breath monitoring, 94–96
Brigham and Women's Hospital (Boston), 12, 132
Brita water filter, 190
Buffalo Health Study, 91
Butler, Robert, 142

caffeine, 125, 126, 139
California Air Resources Board, 185
Calment, Jeanne, 26
calorie counting/restriction, 107, 121, 233
cancer, 50, 65–67, 148, 163, 164
  antibiotics and, 11, 75
  aspirin and, 220
  breast, 11, 75, 202
  cells, 43, 65–66, 148, 181
  depression and, 17
  elevated hs-CRP and, 52
  H. pylori and, 215
  indoor air pollution and, 185
  infections and, 63–64
  leptin and, 101
  low selenium levels and, 206
  magnesium deficiency and, 208
  music and, 184
  polyphenols and, 219
  prostate, 52, 64, 182, 202
  resveratrol and, 219
  smell and, 183
  sunblock and skin, 202
  support groups and, 176
  vitamins and, 202, 205
Candida, 192
Canyon Ranch, 181, 221
carbon dioxide, 85, 88, 127
CARDIA Study (Coronary Artery Risk Development in Young Adults), 162
Carnegie Mellon University, 162
cat scratch fever, 215–216
celiac disease (gluten allergy), 105
cells
  cancer, 43, 65–66, 148, 181
  daughter, 41, 54
  dentritic, 57
  hematogenic, 44
  immune, 32
  lymph, 37
  microglial, 57
  natural killer, 42–43, 92, 181, 182
  red blood, 37, 51, 89
  See also B cells; T cells; white blood cells

Centers for Disease Control and Prevention, 75, 166, 189
cereals, breakfast, 118, 236
chakra system, 181
Chest, 11, 75, 91
chest breathing, 87
Cheyne-Stokes respiration, 94
chlamydia, 215, 216
Chlamydia pneumoniae, 64
chromium, 211–212, 222, 223, 224
chronic infections, 214–219
  See also infections
Chronobiology, 183
chronotherapy, 148
Cipro, 125
Circulation, 15, 127, 143
clavicular breathing, 86–87, 96
Clinical Research in Cardiology, 150
Coccidioides, 192
cockroaches, 194–195
cognitive behavioral therapy, 171
Cohen, Marc, 163
Cohen, Sheldon, 162
communications systems, 47–48
complement system, 45–47, 73
Complete Book of Food Counts, The (Netzer), 121
ConsumerLab.com, 200
C-reactive protein (CRP) blood test. See CRP levels
cribriform plate, 182–183
Crimmins, Eileen, 18, 63
Crohn's disease, 65
CRP levels, 7–8, 31, 57, 59, 60, 71, 72, 91, 111, 221–222, 224
  air pollution and, 9, 185
  anger/hostility and, 15, 70
  anxiety and, 16
  aspirin and, 220
  birth weight and, 10, 179
  depression and, 70
  DHA (docosahexaenoic acid) and, 113
  eating and, 14, 105–106
  exercise and, 10, 143, 144
  fiber and, 114
  heart arrhythmias and, 147
  heart rate variability (HRV) and, 93
  immune activation and, 50–51, 53
  impaired lung function and, 62
  infections and, 216
  insomnia and, 132
  L-carnitine and, 209
  love and, 167
  minerals and, 205

CRP levels (*cont.*)
  physical injury and, 61
  rhythmic movement and, 145, 152
  rowing and, 156
  selenium and, 206
  sleep and, 17, 62, 127–128
  smoking and, 8
  statin medications and, 220
  vitamins and, 15, 201, 204, 205
cruciferous vegetables, 114, 116, 209
Cryptococcus, 192
curcuminoids, 218
cyanosis, 89
cyclosporine, 220
cytokines, 47–48, 51, 56–57, 73, 211, 223
  aspirin and, 220
  cancer and, 67
  chromium picolinate and, 211, 212
  cockroaches and, 194
  exercise and, 143, 144
  genes and, 68
  impaired lung function and, 62
  music and, 184
  narcolepsy and, 132
  sleep and, 129, 130
  zinc and, 207

Dalai Lama, 173
dance. *See* rhythmic movement
daughter cells, 41, 54
DC Water and Sewer Authority, 189
death, causes of, 50
dehumidifiers, 195
delta waves, 127–128, 130
dendritic cells, 57
depression, 69, 70, 71
  aromatherapy and, 183
  exercise and, 145
  healing-touch therapy and, 181
  heart rate variability (HRV) and, 93
  insomnia and, 132
  UltraLongevity quiz and, 16–17
  vitamin D deficiency and, 202
DHA (docosahexaenoic acid), 113, 199
diabetes, 5, 17, 52, 224
  chromium picolinate and, 211
  exercise and, 143
  food allergies and, 105
  leptin and, 101
  lipoic acid and, 211
  magnesium deficiency and, 207–208
  resveratrol and, 219
  vitamins and, 202, 205

diaphragm, 87
diet. *See* eating
digestion, 106, 109, 112–113
DNA, 42, 65, 109, 181
Duke University's Behavior Sciences
    Department, 15, 70
dust mites, 195

eating, 60, 82, 99–123, 227, 228, 229,
    233–237
  calorie counting/restriction, 107, 121, 233
  digestion, 109, 112–113
  elimination diets, 110–111
  emotions and, 103–105, 117
  environment, 108–109, 117
  food allergies, 104–105
  guidelines for eating in/out, 117–123
  hunger and, 100–101, 104–105, 117
  immune-friendly foods, 115–116
  meal plan, 233–237. *See also* RECIPES
  patterns, 101–103, 107–108, 116
  quantity of food, 105–108
  sleep and, 139
  UltraLongevity quiz and, 14
  what to eat, 113–115
  See also weight
edema, 36
electroencephalograph (EEG), 92, 127
elimination diets, 110–111
elliptical trainers, 155
emotions, 68–71, 85, 102, 103–105, 117, 162
emphysema, 91, 94
Enbrel, 47
Endocrine Journal, 144
endorphins, 184
enhancing immune system
  chronic infections and, 214–219
  medications and, 220–221
  taking action for, 221–225
  See also supplements
environment, 178–198
  air and, 184–187
  clean, 189–192
  home, 179–180, 192–194
  household allergens, 192–194
  radon home test, 189
  sleep, 135
  smell and, 182–184
  sound and, 184
  taking action for, 195–198
  touch and, 180–182
  water and, 188–189
  work, 187

Index

Environmental Health Perspectives, 191, 192
Environmental Protection Agency (EPA),
    188–189
enzymes, 56, 57
eosinophils, 44
EPA (eicosapentaenoic acid), 199
Epidemiology, 12, 167
Epstein-Barr virus, 64
eternacept (Enbrel), 220
European Heart Journal, 93
exercise, 9–10, 60, 96, 142, 143–144, 227,
    228
    See also rhythmic movement
exhalation (or expiratory) plateau, 90, 91,
    95
exhalation phase, of breathing, 90, 91, 95
Extreme Makeover: Home Edition, 180
Eye Movement Desensitization and
    Reprocessing, 72

Fabricius, 38
faucet-mount systems, 191
fiber, 114–115, 212–213, 222, 223, 224, 233,
    234
fibroblasts, 56
filtration, 186–187, 190–191, 197
Finch, Caleb, 18, 63
fish, 113–114, 115, 120, 202, 235
fish oils, 199–200, 222, 223, 224, 228, 229
flavonoids, 210
flossing, UltraLongevity quiz and, 12
Fountain of Youth, 3–4, 142
Frankl, Viktor, 173
free radicals, 47, 56, 57
French paradox, 109
Fulford, Robert, 84

Galen, 63
Gallo, Linda, 166
GALT (gut-associated lymphoid tissues), 45
genes, 26
genetic testing, 68–69
genistein, 218–219
ghrelin, 100
Gibran, Kahlil, 173
giraffe dance, 151
Glasgow University, 179
glomerulonephritis, 192
glutathione, 208–209
granzyme (exogenous serine protease), 43
Greek mythology, 149
grocery stores, 235
Groundhog Day, 174

Gunaratana, Bhante H., 84
gut, 45, 72–73, 74, 75, 106, 147, 212–213

Hahnemann School of Medicine
    (Philadelphia), 64
Hanh, Thich Nhat, 173
Harvard Dental School, 12
Harvard Medical School, 51, 132
healing touch, 181–182
Health Psychology, 166
Healthy Women Study, 166
heart arrhythmias, 147, 150
heart disease
    air pollution and, 185
    antibiotics and, 10
    coronary artery disease, 63, 166
    depression and, 16, 17
    emotions and, 70
    exercise and, 144
    heart attacks, 52, 63, 93, 206, 210, 220
    hostility and, 162
    immune activation and, 51
    leptin and, 101
    magnesium deficiency and, 207–208
    resveratrol and, 219
    rheumatic, 64
    sleep and, 133
    stress cardiomyopathy, 166
    vitamins and, 202, 205
    Whipple's disease and, 215
    white blood cells and, 144
heart rate variability (HRV), 92–93
Helen Willis Neuroscience Center (University
    of California, Berkeley), 150
Helicobacter pylori, 53–54, 63, 64
hematogenic cells, 44
hemoglobin, 89
HEPA (high-efficiency particulate air) filters,
    186–187, 193, 195, 196, 197
high blood pressure. *See* blood pressure
highly sensitive CRP test (hs-CRP), 51–52
hiking, 158–159, 176
Hinduism, 149
hip fractures, 61–62
hip/waist measurement, UltraLongevity quiz
    and, 11–12
Histoplasma, 192
HIV (human immunodeficiency virus), 42, 43,
    49, 76, 125, 181
home environment, 179–180, 192–194
hormones, 100, 147
hostility. *See* anger/hostility
H. pylori, 214–215, 216

Index

Human Exposure to Chemicals (Centers for
Disease Control's Third National Report
on), 189–190
Human Genome Project, 68–69
Humira, 47
humor, UltraLongevity quiz and, 13
hunger, 100–101, 104–105, 117
hygiene hypothesis, 76–77
hyperventilation, 88
hypoxia, 62

immune-suppressing medication, 49
immune system, 4–6, 23–48
ALTs (associated lymphoid tissues) and, 45
B cells and, 38–41
bone marrow and, 33–34
communications systems and, 47–48
complement system and, 45–47
hematogenic cells and, 44
how it works, 23–32
lymphatic system and, 35–37
spleen and, 35
T cells and, 41–44
thymus and, 34–35
white blood cells and, 37
See also breathing; eating; enhancing immune
system; environment; immune system,
overactive; love; quiz, UltraLongevity;
rhythmic movement; sleep
immune system, overactive, 49–78
aging and, 54–55, 58–59
antibiotics and, 74–75
cancer and, 65–67
CRP test and, 51–52
emotions and, 68–71
genetic testing and, 68–69
hygiene hypothesis and, 76–77
hypoxia and, 62
infections and, 63–65
invaders and, 55–57
patients' stories and, 53–54, 58–60, 71–72
physical injury and, 61–62
See also immune system
immunoglobulin A, 182
Imuran, 220
incentive spirometer, 97
infections, 49, 50, 53–54, 63–65, 76
See also chronic infections
infliximab (Remicade), 220
inhalation (or inspiratory) plateau, of
breathing, 90, 95
inhalation phase, of breathing, 90, 95
insomnia, 132–133, 140, 183

interferons, 47
interleukin-1, 132
interleukin-6, 206, 207
chromium picolinate and, 211
eating and, 14
music and, 184
sleep apnea and, 129
interleukin-8, 194
interleukins, 47, 59, 130
International Journal of Cardiology, 143
International Journal of Neuroscience, 181
International Journal of Sports Medicine, 145
International Longevity Center, 142
International Psychogeriatrics, 150
interval training, 159
inversion tables, 198

JAMA, 61–62, 69, 75, 162, 182
James H. Quillen College of Medicine (East
Tennessee State University), 144
jellyfish, 28–29
jogging, 157, 159
Journal of Alternative and Complementary
Medicine, 92
Journal of Cardiovascular Electrophysiology, 93
Journal of Circulation, 205
Journal of Clinical Endocrinology &
Metabolism, 129
Journal of Epidemiology and Community Health, 11
Journal of Pediatrics, 143
Journal of the American College of Cardiology,
12, 17
Journal of the American Medical Association
(JAMA), 8
journals, 172
jumping rope, 157
Just Tomatoes, Etc.!, 119
Just Vegetable Munchies, 119

Korean study, 150
!Kung tribe (of Kalahari desert), 151

LaLanne, Jack, 142
L-arginine, 210, 224
Las Vegas roach traps, 194–195, 196
lavender, 183
L-carnitine, 209–210, 224
lead, 189, 190
leptin, 100–101, 144, 211, 223
Levaquin, 125
Life Sciences, 184
life span, 26–27
lighting, 180

Index

limonene, 214
Lipitor, 60, 220
lipoic acid, 210–211, 224
Lord of the Rings, The, 180
love, 83, 161–177, 226, 227
  acceptance and, 163–164
  as daily event, 168–170
  interpersonal, 165–168
  of nature, 161, 164–165
  taking action for, 170–177
  UltraLongevity quiz and, 12–13
  for yourself, 167
Love Is the Killer App (Sanders), 173
lung diseases, 91, 94, 215
Luvox, 125
lycopene, 219
Lyme disease, 215, 216
lymphatic system, 35–37
lymph nodes, 36–37
lymphocytes, 37, 41

macrophages (MPs), 56–57, 166
  B cells and, 39–40, 40–41
  cancer and, 66–67
  complement system and, 46
  GALT (gut-associated lymphoid tissues)
    and, 45
  smoking and, 8
magnesium, 207–208, 222, 224
Man's Search for Meaning (Frankl), 173
mantras, 138, 174–175
martial arts, 158
massage, 14, 60, 137, 181, 197
Mayeroff, Milton, 173
Mayo Clinic, 127
Mechanisms of Aging and Development, 55
Medical Science Monitor, 184
medications, 220–221, 222
meditation, 136, 151–152, 158, 198, 226
memory, 29, 38–39, 54–55
mercury, 191–192, 200
metastasis, 67
methotrexate, 220
microglial cells (microglia), 57
MIDSPAN Family Study, 10, 179
migraines, 193, 194, 207–208, 225
milk thistle (silymarin), 225
mindful breathing, 92
Mindfulness in Plain English (Gunaratana), 84
minerals, 205–208
molds, 192–194, 196
Molecules of Emotion (Pert), 71
monocytes, 44

Mount Sinai Hospital (Manhattan), 142
movies, 174
MRSA (methicillin-resistant Staphylococcus
    aureus), 75
mucous membranes, 148
multiple sclerosis, 65, 202, 211
muscle-relaxation exercise, 136
music, 60, 184
  breathing and, 98
  healing effects of, 149–150
  home environment and, 196, 197
  jumping rope and, 157
  pain and, 150
  Parkinson's disease patients and, 146
  rowing and, 156
  UltraLongevity quiz and, 17–18
myocarditis, 65

N-acetyl cysteine (NAC), 209, 225
narcolepsy, 132
National Health and Nutrition Examination
    Survey, 143
National Institute of Allergy and Infectious
    Diseases, 194
National Institute of Environmental Health
    Sciences, 194
National Institute of Health, 71
National Institute on Aging, 63
natural killer cells (NKs), 42–43, 92, 181,
    182
nature, 161, 164–165
Netzer, Corrine, 121
Neurobiology of Aging, 64
NeuroImmunoModulation, 182
Neuroscience Research, 92
neutrophils, 44
New England Journal of Medicine, 16, 166
night terrors, 131
Nike + iPod Sport Kit, 157
nitric oxide, 47
non-REM sleep, 127, 131
Nurses Health Study, 133
nuts, 114, 116

obesity, 102, 126, 133, 143, 144, 202
  See also weight
obestatin, 100
oils, 114, 122–123
  See also fish oils
olfactory nerve, 183
Omega Man, The, 165
On Caring (Mayeroff), 173
Organic Just Fruit, 119

Index

osteoporosis
  depression and, 16
  magnesium deficiency and, 207–208
  vitamin D deficiency and, 202

panic attacks, 85–86, 87
Parkinson's disease, 146
Pauling, Linus, 203
PCBs (polychlorinated biphenyls), 200
PCE (perchloroethylene), 185
Peace Is Every Step (Hanh), 173
Pediatric Nursing, 18
pedometers, 153, 157, 228, 229
Penn State University, 129
perforin, 43
Pert, Candace, 71
pets, 13, 137, 172
physical injury, 61–62
phytonutrients, 218–219
Picture Perfect Weight Loss (Shapiro), 121
pitchers/carafes, 190, 197
pizzica tarantata, 151
plaque, 56–57, 69, 162
pollution. *See* air pollution
polychlorinated biphenyls (PCBs), 200
polymorphonuclear cells. *See* neutrophils
polypeptides, 109
polyphenols, 219
Ponce de León, Juan, 3
Pravachol, 220
prayer, 164
Pressman, Sarah, 162
probiotics (symbiotic/desirable bacteria), 74,
  77, 114, 212–213, 216–218, 224, 227, 229
Prophet, The (Gibran), 173
prostatitis, 215, 216
proteins, 43, 47–48, 57, 109–110, 112,
  208–209
psoriasis, 206
Psychiatry, 145
Psychological Bulletin, 162
Psychosomatic Medicine, 15, 70, 146, 166
psychotherapy, 171
pulse, 92
pursed-lip breathing, 89
pyrogens, 47, 220

quercetin, 210
quiz, UltraLongevity, 7–19

radon, 185, 189
reading, 173–174

RECIPES
breads
  Whole Wheat Flaxseed Bread,
    250–251
  Whole Wheat Risotto Bread, 272–273
breakfast
  Banana Berry Smoothie, 276
  Blueberry Pancakes, 270–271
  Chicken Sausage, 264
  Egg White Omelet with Vegetables, 238
  Multigrain French Toast, 255
  Yogurt with Fruit and Nuts, 250
desserts
  Apple Strudel, 268–269
  Banana Yogurt Smoothie, 249
  Cranberry Apple Betty, 244
  Maple Orange Flan, 262–263
  Pear Crisp, 275
dressings
  Balsamic Dijon Dressing, 247–248
  Ginger Soy Dressing, 266
  Sesame Ginger Dressing, 278–279
  Thousand Island Dressing, 273
main dishes
  Asian Cabbage Rolls with Mongolian
    BBQ Sauce, 242
  Bean and Vegetable Quesadillas, 251–252
  Cantonese Tempeh Stir-Fry, 281–282
  Cardamom Grilled Chicken with Mango
    Lime Sauce, 261–262
  Chicken Fajitas, 279–280
  Grilled Salmon with Mongolian BBQ
    Sauce, 268
  Grilled Vegetable Strudel with Tomato
    Olive Sauce, 282–283
  Horseradish-Crusted Salmon with
    Cranberry Dill Catsup, 253–254
  Olive Oil, Parmesan, and Black Pepper
    Pasta, 275
  Raspberry Cornish Hen, 248–249
  Southwest Grilled Chicken Quesadillas
    with Avocado Salad, 246–247
  Tempeh Fajitas, 285
  Tilapia with Tomato Orange Salsa, 258
  Vegetarian Bean Chili, 284–285
salads
  Asian Duck Salad with Ginger Soy
    Dressing, 266–267
  Carrot and Raisin Salad, 274
  Curried Tofu Salad in Pita, 282
  Kamut Salad with Dried Cranberries,
    271–272

Index

Mixed Green Salad with Sesame Ginger
Dressing, 278–279
Sole with Lemon Grass–Red Bell Pepper
Salad, 243
Spinach Salad with Pecans, 247
Waldorf Salad, 260
sandwiches
California Turkey Wrap, 277
Cranberry Chicken Wrap, 256–257
Grilled Vegetable Wrap, 240–241
Open-Faced Turkey Reuben, 272
sauces and relishes
Guacamole, 280
Mango Lime Sauce, 261–262
Maple Caramel Sauce, 262–263
Mediterranean Pasta Sauce, 257
Mongolian BBQ Sauce, 242–243
Tartar Sauce, 259
Tomato Olive Sauce, 283–284
side dishes
Baked Sweet Potatoes, 248
Gingered Spiced Carrots, 252–253
Mashed Sweet Potatoes, 261
Roasted Acorn Squash, 274
Steamed Vegetable Basket, 257, 267
snacks
Canyon Ranch Trail Bars (Gluten-Free), 241
soups
Chicken Stock for, 265–266
Cream of Broccoli Soup, 245–246
Mulligatawny Soup, 265
Spring Pea Soup, 256
Tortilla Soup, 239–240
Vegetable Stock for, 240
red blood cells, 37, 51, 89
Remicade, 47
REM sleep, 127–128, 130
RESPeRATE, 98
resveratrol, 219
reverse-osmosis systems, 191
Reyataz, 125
rheumatoid arthritis, 65, 76, 164, 181
rhythmic movement, 82–83, 141–160
built-in rhythms, 146–149
power of, 145–146
rhythm and dance, 149–152
taking action for, 153–160
See also exercise
Ridker, Paul, 51, 52
rowing, 156, 159
Royal Melbourne Institute of Technology,
163

Sanders, Tim, 173
SCID (severe combined immunodeficiency
disease), 179
Science, 18, 150
sedimentation (sed) rate, 51, 61, 111, 223
selegiline (deprenyl), 211
selenium, 114, 205–206, 222
serotonin, 103
sexuality, 12, 147, 182
Shapiro, Howard, 121
siblings, 11
sick building syndrome (SBS), 186, 187
sighing, 97–98
silymarin, 218
sinus infections, 215
sleep, 82, 124–140, 226, 229
disorders, 125, 131, 132
immune system and, 129–132
importance of high quality, 126–129
insomnia, 132–133, 140, 183
medications, 126
taking action for, 133–140
UltraLongevity quiz and, 17
sleep apnea, 62, 127–128, 131
sleeping sickness, 130
smell, 182–184, 196
smoking, 8
social connectedness, 167
sound, 184, 197
Southern Medical Journal, 164
spinal fusion, 152
spleen, 33, 35
sports, competitive, 158
Stachybotrys, 193
Stanford Center for Narcolepsy Research, 132
statin medications, 220
steroids, 49, 53, 111
Strahlentherapie und Onkologie, 164
stress
acceptance and, 164
aromatherapy and, 183
eating and, 108
hearing and, 184
music and, 149
sleep and, 125, 131
stress cardiomyopathy, 166
stroke, 51, 77
aspirin and, 220
depression and, 17
elevated hs-CRP and, 52
infections and, 63
vitamin B12 and, 205

297

Index

substance abuse, 125–126
sulforaphane, 114
supplements, 60, 142, 199–214, 222, 227, 228
  chromium, 211–212, 222, 223, 224
  fiber, 212–213
  fish oils, 199–200, 222, 224, 228, 229
  glutathione, 208–209
  L-arginine, 210
  L-carnitine, 209–210
  lipoic acid, 210–211
  minerals, 205–208
  N-acetyl cysteine (NAC), 209, 225
  quercetin, 210
  vitamins, 201–205
  water, 213–214
support groups, 176
sweeteners, 236
swimming, 98, 145, 155, 159

Tagamet, 125
tai chi, 151, 158
tap dancing, 157
TCE (trichloroethylene), 185
T cells, 39, 41–44, 57
  GALT (gut-associated lymphoid tissues)
    and, 45
  hearing and, 184
  lymph nodes and, 37
  thymus and, 34, 35
tennis, 141, 151, 158
therapy, 171
theta rhythms, 150
thioctic acid. *See* lipoic acid
third world countries, 50
Thorax, 62, 91
thymus, 34–35
TNF-alpha, 62, 91, 129, 130, 132, 144, 207, 211
TNFs (tumor necrosis factors), 47
touch, 180–182
trance, 150–151
trypanosome, 130
tuberculosis, 75, 91
tumors, 65–66
turmeric powder, 218

under-the-sink systems, 191
United Nations Children's Fund, 188
United States Geological Survey, 188
University of California (San Francisco), 64

University of Southern California School of
  Gerontology, 63
USDA Nutrient Database, 223
U.S. Department of Agriculture, 121
U.S. Environmental Protection Agency, 185
USP label (United States Pharmacopeia),
  200, 201
uveitis, 53–54, 215

valley fever, 192
ventilation, 186
viruses, 42–43
vitamins, 14–15, 60, 67, 201–205, 222, 223,
  224, 227, 229
VOCs (volatile organic compounds), 185,
  190
VRE (vancomycin-resistant *Enterococcus*), 75

walking, 152–154, 228, 229
Warwick Medical School (England), 133
water, 188–189, 190, 197, 213–214, 227, 228,
  236
weight, 82, 211–212, 223, 224
  birth, 10, 18, 179
  calorie counting and, 121
  exercise and, 143
  sleep and, 126, 127
  UltraLongevity quiz and, 7–8
  See also obesity
What Happy People Know (Baker), 173
Whipple's disease, 215
white blood cells, 56, 59, 71, 91, 148, 223
  chromium picolinate and, 211
  exercise and, 143, 144
  heart rate variability (HRV) and, 93
  hematogenic cells and, 44
  immune system and, 37
  impaired lung function and, 62
  infections and, 216
  physical injury and, 61
  smoking and, 8
  See also T cells
white-coat high blood pressure, 86
Wilkes University (Pennsylvania), 182
work environment, 187
World Health Organization, 186, 188

zinc, 206–207, 222, 224
Zocor, 220
Zyflo, 125